I0765487

Lessons From the Body

Matthew Tamer

Fixed Point Press

Lessons From the Body. Copyright © 2026 by Matthew Tamer. All rights reserved. Published by Fixed Point Press. Please spread the contents of this book far and wide to anyone who would benefit from the words on these pages. Borrow, plagiarize, and do whatever you will. If you have the courtesy to cite this book as your source when using content, it would be greatly appreciated.

First Edition

Designed by Matthew Tamer
Images generated in collaboration with ChatGPT

ISBN: 979-8-9946670-0-2 (Paperback)
ISBN: 979-8-9946670-2-6 (Hardcover)
ISBN: 979-8-9946670-1-9 (E-Book)

To my boy: Thank you for teaching me so much more than I
could ever hope to teach you.

You are my best friend in the whole world.

I love you today and every day.

You make me so happy.

I am so proud of you.

Pinky promise. Deal!

Table of Contents

Introduction

Throughout life, I have noticed that the same lessons appear again and again—sometimes in relationships, sometimes in failure, sometimes in the quiet signals of the body itself. Long before we can name what is happening, something inside us already knows. It tightens. It resists. It adapts.

This book is an invitation to look inward—not for judgment or diagnosis, but for wisdom.

This book uses accessible reflections on the body's systems to explore deeper truths our conscious minds may have forgotten. There will be moments of science along the way, but this is not a textbook, nor is it an exercise in memorization. My hope is not that you retain every detail, but that you recognize something familiar—that you remember the lessons your body has been teaching you all along.

Life has a way of narrowing our focus. Pain, responsibility, and loss can obscure parts of ourselves we once knew well. But by learning what you are made of, you may begin to remember who you are—and who you are still becoming.

Thank you for joining me on this journey, my friend.

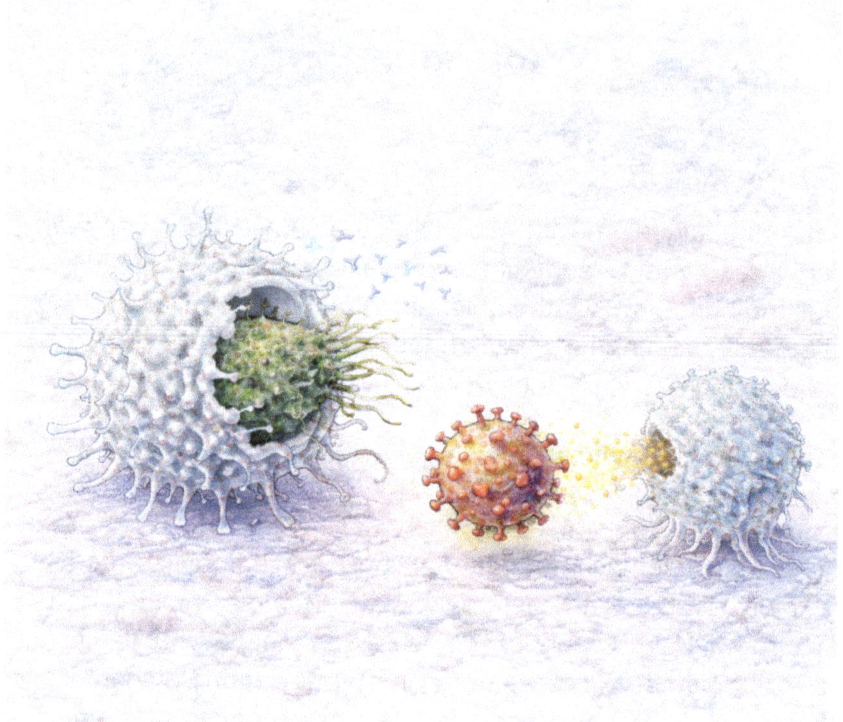

Immune System:

Protection Without Destruction

Immune System: Protection Without Destruction

Most of us do not set out to become guarded.

We learn it slowly—through disappointment, loss, betrayal, or fear. Something hurts, and the body remembers. We become more watchful. More selective. We learn to anticipate harm before it arrives. Over time, this vigilance begins to feel like wisdom. After all, protection is how we survive.

But there is a quiet cost to living this way.

When protection becomes constant, the body never rests. We remain braced even in moments of safety. Neutral experiences begin to feel threatening. What once helped us endure slowly begins to limit our capacity to live.

This is not a failure of character. It is not weakness. It is the predictable result of a system doing its best to keep us safe after injury.

The immune system exists for this very purpose.

In the human body, the immune system is responsible for one of the most delicate tasks in existence: discernment. It must constantly decide what belongs and what does not—what can be welcomed and what must be addressed. This decision-making happens relentlessly, at every moment, without conscious effort. And when it works well, we never notice it at all.

The immune system is not aggressive by nature. It is thoughtful. Its goal is not destruction, but preservation—maintaining balance within a complex and vulnerable organism. Health depends not on eliminating all threats, but on responding appropriately to them.

To understand how this works, it helps to look at the system itself.

The immune system is a vast network of specialized cells, tissues, and signaling molecules working together to maintain homeostasis—the body's internal equilibrium. Like a well-coordinated public safety system, it relies on communication, memory, and restraint.

When a threat enters the body—such as a virus, bacterium, or abnormal cell—early responders move in quickly. Cells like macrophages and dendritic cells identify the intruder and attempt to contain it locally. At the same time, they release chemical signals that alert the broader immune network, much like an alarm notifying emergency services.

These signals travel to nearby lymph nodes, where information is processed and shared. T cells are activated and multiplied, forming a coordinated response team. Some of these cells direct the response, ensuring it remains targeted. Others carry out the work of neutralizing infected or damaged cells. Once the threat has been resolved, the system stands down.

Importantly, this response is temporary.

The immune system is designed to act decisively—and then rest.

Discernment, however, is learned.

Early in life, immune cells are exposed to countless signals as they learn what belongs within the body and what does not. Some responses are excessive. Others are delayed. But over time, through feedback and correction, the system becomes more precise. Memory cells are formed after successful responses, allowing future threats to be handled more efficiently. Regulatory mechanisms quiet reactions that are no longer needed.

Health does not require perfection. It requires adaptability.

An immune system that never responds becomes vulnerable. One that never quiets becomes dangerous. Balance is maintained only through continual reassessment.

When this discernment is lost, the consequences can be profound.

Autoimmune diseases offer a clear example. In these conditions, the immune system misidentifies healthy tissue as a threat. The response that once protected the body now harms it. The system is not malicious—it is confused. Past learning has been misapplied.

Celiac disease illustrates this clearly. In individuals with this condition, gluten is mistakenly identified as a dangerous invader. Each exposure triggers an immune cascade that damages the lining of the small intestine. Over time, inflammation impairs nutrient absorption, leading to fatigue, anemia, bone weakness, and widespread systemic effects.

What makes this process tragic is not its intent, but its accuracy. The immune system responds exactly as it was trained to respond—just to the wrong signal.

A similar pattern often unfolds in our emotional lives.

Many of us carry internal alarm systems shaped by past injury. Relationships end. Trust is broken. Safety is compromised. The mind and body learn quickly, storing these experiences as reference points. Over time, those memories begin to influence how we interpret the present.

Neutral interactions feel charged. Silence feels threatening. New experiences are scanned for familiar danger. We become exhausted—not because we are weak, but because we are constantly protecting ourselves.

Like an immune system stuck in overdrive, we may begin responding to situations that no longer require defense. Opportunities for connection, growth, and joy are quietly filtered out—not because they are harmful, but because they resemble something that once was.

Here is the wisdom the immune system offers us:

True strength is not found in constant defense, but in wise protection.

There are moments when boundaries are essential, when harm must be recognized and addressed decisively. But not every unfamiliar experience is a threat. Not every discomfort requires retreat. Discernment allows us to respond with precision rather than panic.

Learning this takes time.

Just as immune cells refine their responses through experience and feedback, we learn—slowly—how to differentiate past danger from present possibility. Healing does not mean erasing memory. It means allowing memory to inform without controlling.

This book begins here because protection is often where pain leaves its deepest imprint. And it continues because the body, when listened to, knows how to restore balance.

The immune system does not seek destruction. It seeks belonging.

And so do we.

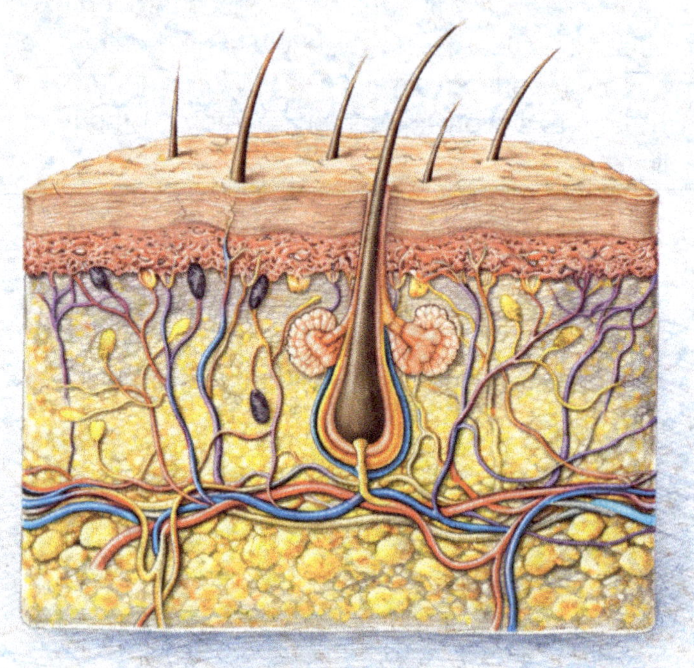

Skin:

Boundaries That Still Allow Connection

Skin: Boundaries That Still Allow Connection

Skin is the first boundary we ever know. Long before language, it teaches us what closeness feels like, what pressure means, and where we end and the world begins. It holds warmth and releases heat. It receives comfort and registers pain. Every moment, it negotiates contact—deciding what may touch us, what must be kept out, and what can safely pass through.

Because of this, skin is not merely a covering. It is a living interface between protection and connection. Too little defense, and we are vulnerable to harm. Too much, and we become isolated, sealed off from the very sensations that make us feel alive. Healthy skin does not exist to block the world—it exists to relate to it wisely.

Our emotional boundaries function much the same way. They are not meant to harden us into distance, nor dissolve us into exposure. They are meant to help us stay present—open enough to connect, firm enough to remain ourselves. Like skin, boundaries that are alive can adapt. They can thicken where protection is needed and soften where trust has been earned.

The body understands this balance intuitively. And if we are willing to listen, it can teach us how to build boundaries that do not cost us connection.

Human skin has two main layers: the epidermis and the dermis. Some of this may sound familiar—remember the childhood quip, "Your epidermis is showing"? The epidermis is the outermost layer, made of several sublayers, or "strata," of cells. It has two main jobs. First, it locks moisture into the lower layers, keeping skin hydrated and flexible enough to handle daily strain. Second, it forms a protective barrier across the body, defending against the outside world. Think of it like the skin of a piece of fruit—the tough, fibrous layer that shields the vulnerable flesh beneath.

The epidermis is often described as a "brick-and-mortar" structure, with each cell acting as a brick held together by fatty mortar. These cells have no blood vessels of their own; only the bottom layer receives nourishment from capillaries in the dermis beneath. Gradually, the bottom cells move upward, maturing into flat, durable cells. By the time they reach the surface, they have lost most internal structure, forming the stratum corneum—a layer of essentially dead cells. This journey takes roughly a month in adults, though it slows with age. At the surface, millions of these cells are shed daily.

This shedding is not a sign of failure—it is evidence of renewal. The epidermis is constantly replacing itself, quietly repairing damage accumulated through daily exposure. Most of this regeneration occurs while we sleep, when cellular turnover accelerates and resources are redirected toward repair. When sleep is disrupted or stress is chronic, this process falters. Skin may become dry, inflamed, slow to heal, or more reactive to its environment. What we see on the surface often reflects what is happening beneath it.

The body does not restore itself through force, but through rhythm. Protection is maintained not by rigidity, but by continuous renewal.

The dermis is the second layer of skin—far more alive than the epidermis above. Made of connective tissue, it provides strength and elasticity through substances like collagen and hyaluronan. Hair follicles begin in this layer before pushing up through the epidermis. Sweat glands, also found here, help regulate body temperature—athletes, take note and be grateful! Sebaceous, or oil, glands lubricate skin and hair while keeping surrounding cells supple and resilient, which contributes to elasticity. The dermis also contains numerous nerve endings, giving us our sense of touch and temperature—one of the main ways we connect with the world.

This balance between protection and exposure is not unique to skin. A useful analogy for the epidermis and dermis is a smartphone. The epidermis is like the glass screen: we see and interact with it, but it is not alive without the layers beneath. The dermis is the motherboard and internal structures, constantly processing and transmitting information while being protected. Both layers must work in harmony. The screen only displays what happens underneath; the motherboard can accomplish so much, yet it is vulnerable to the outside world. Neither layer can function without the other—they rely on one another and must coexist in balance.

But what if this balance were disrupted? If the epidermis thickened to block every external threat, the dermis beneath could not function properly. Oil glands could struggle to keep the skin supple, and the skin itself could become stiff and brittle. Temperature regulation would falter. Most importantly, one would lose touch with the world—literally. Like a gloved hand desperately trying to send a text. Skin would become calloused and numb; a warm hug might lose its magic, and holding hands with a loved one could feel lifeless.

What if the opposite happened, and the epidermis became too thin? The risk of injury would rise sharply, with outside forces penetrating vulnerable inner layers. Hydration could escape as vital elements leak from the skin unchecked. Too much body heat might be lost, causing chills and rigors. Even gentle stimuli could feel intense. Anxiety and stress could easily follow. In short, healthy skin depends on a delicate balance between protection and vulnerability—neither can exist without the other. And when these boundaries are repeatedly violated or held too tightly, the nervous system often bears the cost—remaining tense, vigilant, and slow to trust the world it is meant to interpret.

Here is the wisdom skin offers us: boundaries can be healthy. They protect the sensitive, emotional parts of ourselves—but balance is essential. Boundaries should not be so thick that we become like calloused skin, unable to feel. Protection may feel comforting, but too much comes at the cost of life-giving connection. Boundaries are not walls—they are living systems, flexible and adaptable. Nor should they be too thin or absent, leaving us exposed to constant harm. People-pleasing often stems from this vulnerability, with guilt and shame arising even from saying a simple "no." Healthy boundaries are not just beneficial—they are essential to living intentionally. Like skin, they allow us to remain safe while still experiencing intimacy, connection, and care—the things that make life feel real.

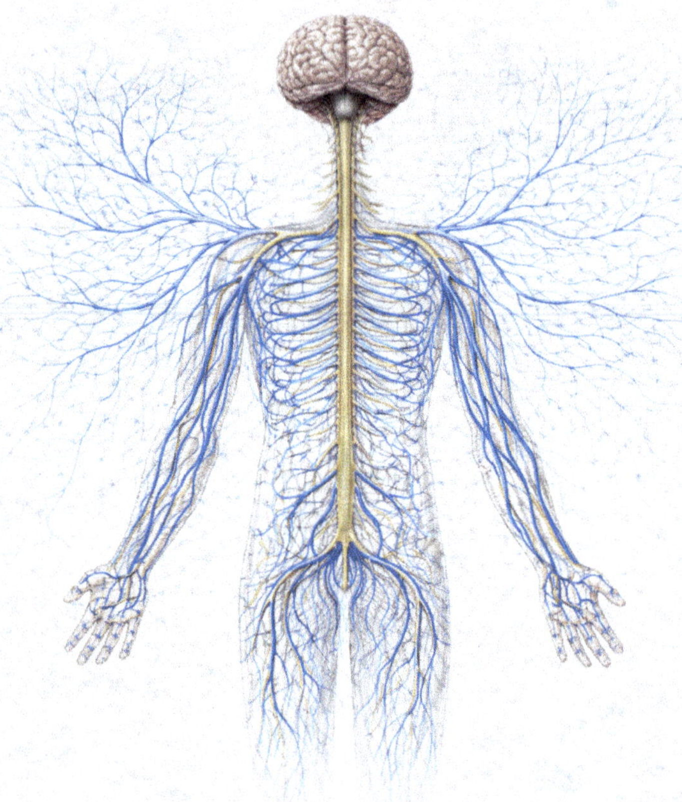

Nervous System:

Responding, Not Living in Alarm

Nervous System: Responding, Not Living in Alarm

Before we ever learn the language of stress or trauma, the nervous system speaks to us in sensation. A tight chest before a conversation. A shallow breath that never quite deepens. The constant hum of vigilance that makes rest feel unsafe and stillness feel suspicious. For many of us, this state becomes so familiar that we mistake it for personality.

The nervous system exists to keep us alive. It scans for danger, prepares us to act, and mobilizes energy when a threat appears. This capacity is not a flaw—it is a gift. But a system designed for short bursts of protection can become overwhelmed when it is asked to stay on high alert indefinitely.

When alarm becomes a lifestyle rather than a response, the body pays the price. Muscles remain tense. Thoughts race. Emotions feel louder and less controllable. And even in moments of safety, the system struggles to stand down. What protects us in moments of danger can quietly exhaust us when it becomes a way of life.

The nervous system was never meant to trap us in fear. It was meant to help us respond—then return. To act when necessary, and to rest when danger has passed. Learning the difference between responding to life and living in alarm is not about eliminating fear; it is about teaching the body that safety can exist again.

The body already knows how to do this. The question is whether we will help it remember.

Just as skin thickens or thins in response to injury, the nervous system adapts to what it endures—sometimes protecting us, sometimes exhausting us in the process.

Like the electrical wiring behind walls, the nervous system is a network of interconnected cells and tissues that coordinates all of the body's activities. By transmitting and receiving signals, the nervous system controls both essential and nonessential functions. These responsibilities divide the nervous system into two main parts.

The first is the autonomic nervous system, which manages essential, nonconscious functions. These include maintaining heart rate, breathing rate, and digestion. All of the most vital processes for living fall into this category, and the body has a remarkable way of regulating them while leaving the brain free to focus on other endeavors. Could you imagine if you had to consciously concentrate on every breath or every heartbeat? We would become a population of stagnant, lifeless people focused solely on survival.

The second part is the voluntary (or somatic) nervous system, which controls conscious movement, such as kicking a soccer ball or using a fork to eat. This portion of the nervous system connects to skeletal muscle and allows us to contract or relax parts of our bodies at will. While it is not strictly necessary for survival, it offers tremendous quality of life. Imagine how dull life would be without intentional movement. We would all be sentenced to a sedentary existence—no cooking, painting, rock climbing, or so much more. Instead, we get to chase our passions in a world full of incredible things to discover. Behind every unbelievable feat is a finely tuned somatic nervous system operating at high efficiency.

Some protective responses are so fast they bypass conscious thought entirely—designed to act before we can decide. When these reflex defenses are unable to resolve a perceived threat quickly, prolonged stress can activate the body's fight-or-flight response. In this state, hormones flood the body and part of the autonomic nervous system kicks into overdrive. Focus sharpens, alertness increases, and nonessential functions like digestion are temporarily shut down. Muscles tense, pain perception decreases, and physical limits may be pushed beyond the norm. There are even documented cases of extraordinary strength during fight-or-flight—individuals lifting cars or heavy objects to rescue others. It is an incredible gift.

So why don't our bodies remain in this state more often? Couldn't we simply harness this hidden potential by stressing ourselves? Unfortunately, the truth is more sobering. Like an immune system that cannot stand down, a nervous system stuck in alarm begins to do more harm than good. Survival mode is meant for emergencies, not everyday life. Like faulty electrical wiring in a house, everything may appear functional on the surface—while unseen damage quietly builds behind the walls. When we remain under chronic stress, the consequences can be debilitating. Long-term effects may include high blood pressure and heart disease, anxiety, depression, digestive issues, and sleep disturbances. Our bodies also lose capacity to engage the somatic nervous system—the system that enables joy, creativity, and purpose. As quality of life declines, stress compounds, creating a self-sustaining cycle of mental and physical strain.

Here is the wisdom offered by the nervous system: we are not meant to live in a constant state of alarm. While modern life contains fewer physical threats than ever before—most people are no longer hunting and gathering while watching for predators—we have traded those dangers for internal and existential ones.

Many of us spend our days working demanding, unfulfilling jobs, sometimes multiple at once, simply to sustain patterns of overconsumption. Our relationships suffer as we live increasingly isolated lives, exchanging true connection for shallow digital interaction. We approach situations as though they require a fight-or-flight response, overreacting to even the smallest transgressions. Without meaningful connection, we feel lost and alone—anxious and depressed. Physical health deteriorates, and the underlying causes feel overwhelming to address. This is the modern version of survival mode. This is what chronic stress looks like.

And many of us have lived there for years.

A nervous system in survival mode is not resting—it is constantly interpreting. Every interaction is scanned for threat. Every silence is filled with meaning. Neutral events are assigned emotional weight, and the mind becomes exhausted not by action, but by vigilance. Over time, this hyperinterpretation erodes trust—in others, in circumstances, and in oneself. Joy feels unsafe. Stillness feels suspicious. Even rest can provoke anxiety, as though something important is being missed.

This is not a failure of character. It is the predictable outcome of a system that has not been allowed to stand down.

But all is not lost. It *is* possible to reset your internal state, though it requires intention and effort. The first step is simple in concept but challenging in practice: reconnect. Reconnect with others, and reconnect with yourself. Connection provides belonging and a sense of home. Few experiences are as deeply satisfying as being fully known and accepted. Many of us have never taken the time to truly know ourselves. We are taught that goals, milestones, prestige, and money lead to fulfillment, yet the truth is that the people around us often make all the difference. Have you ever experienced something that should have been incredible—a lifelong dream realized—only to have it diminished by someone who complained the entire time? Conversely, do you have a cherished memory of doing absolutely nothing with someone you love, laughing without even knowing why? What made one experience painful and the other joyful? The people. Be intentional about finding your people, and then go deeper in those relationships.

The second step may feel more daunting: change what isn't working. This is rarely straightforward. Some feel trapped in stressful jobs due to financial obligations or health insurance needs. Others remain in painful relationships long past their expiration dates. The solutions may not be immediately clear, and you may not be able to walk away right away—but you *can* take steps. Begin exploring new job opportunities or advocating for meaningful change where you are. Be willing to have difficult conversations within strained relationships and to work collaboratively toward growth, whether together or apart.

Finally, physical movement can be one of the most powerful tools for restoring balance. Gentle activities such as stretching, yoga, or walking can function like a pressure-release valve for the nervous system. Reduce distractions, quiet external stimulation, and focus on your movement and breath. If you can move outdoors, even better. Over time, as your nervous system learns that it is safe to stand down, you may discover something profound: just as a well-wired home allows energy to flow without constant sparks or overloads, a well-regulated nervous system allows you to live with presence, purpose, and ease. In that space, you are no longer merely surviving—you are truly living.

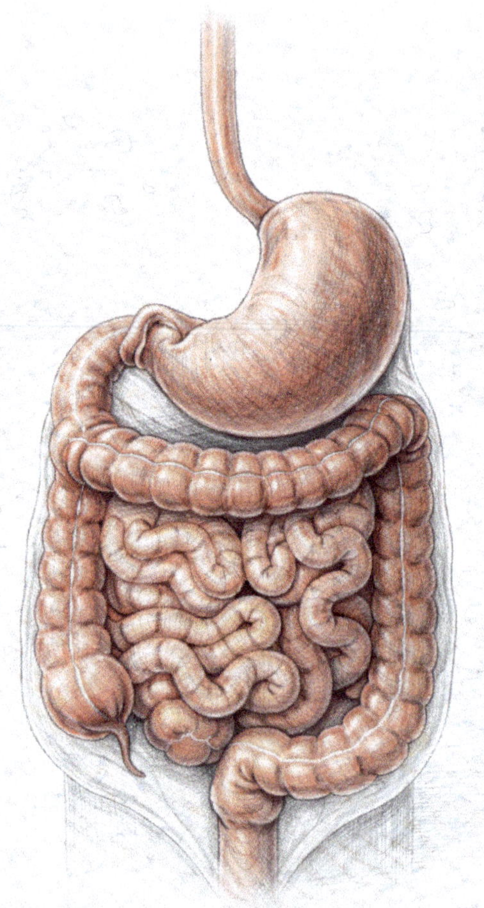

Digestive System:
Choosing What Nourishes

Digestive System: Choosing What Nourishes

The digestive system is one of the first systems we rely on—and one of the few that never stops asking us to choose. From the moment we are born, it performs a quiet, constant act of discernment: deciding what will be taken in, what will be transformed, and what must be released. Without this ongoing refinement, there would be no energy, no growth, no repair—only accumulation and depletion. Like a blacksmith's forge, the digestive system does not simply accept raw material. It subjects everything to heat and process, extracting what can sustain life and discarding what cannot.

The human body is remarkably versatile, capable of deriving value from an astonishing variety of foods. Fruits and vegetables, grains and proteins, salts and fats—all are transformed into the building blocks that sustain life. Somehow, the body knows how to make use of each component. Yet despite this elegance, we are often mindless consumers. We fill ourselves with highly processed foods and chemical additives, then expect the digestive system to sort through the chaos without consequence. To better appreciate its wisdom, we must take a closer look.

Digestion begins in a place we all know well: the mouth. Here, raw material enters the body and is mechanically broken down by teeth and saliva. Blacksmiths use a similar strategy when smelting iron—raw ore is crushed into smaller pieces to increase surface area, allowing heat and chemicals to work more efficiently. In the same way, chewing and saliva prepare food for the chemical processes that follow, increasing efficiency and reducing strain on the system downstream.

From the mouth, food travels to the stomach—the furnace of the digestive system. In a forge, intense heat reduces raw ore to a malleable state, loosening impurities so they can be removed. Additional materials, known as flux, may be added to bind these impurities and separate them from the usable metal. The stomach performs a comparable function. Powerful gastric acids chemically break food down, while enzymes such as gastric lipase begin digesting fats. Strong muscular contractions churn the mixture continuously, ensuring thorough contact between food, acid, and enzymes.

The result of this process is chyme: a thick, semi-liquid mixture prepared for the next stage of refinement. Like molten metal awaiting purification, chyme is not yet useful on its own—but it is ready.

From the stomach, chyme enters the small intestine, where most digestion and nutrient absorption take place. At the beginning of this journey, bile from the liver and enzymes from the pancreas are introduced. Bile assists primarily in fat digestion, while pancreatic enzymes help break down fats, proteins, and carbohydrates. Additional enzymes produced by the intestinal lining further dismantle complex carbohydrates into absorbable components.

As this mixture moves through the small intestine, millions of tiny, finger-like projections called villi line the intestinal walls. These structures dramatically increase surface area and act as selective gatekeepers, absorbing nutrients and water while keeping harmful substances out. Nutrients pass through the villi directly into the bloodstream, where they are transported throughout the body to support energy production, tissue repair, muscle growth, and the creation of new enzymes.

Meanwhile, what cannot be used remains behind. The villi are highly discerning; they must be. Allowing waste or toxins into circulation would compromise the entire system—much like using impure metal in construction. Weakness introduced at the foundation increases the risk of cracks and failure elsewhere. Discernment at this stage is not optional; it is essential.

Absorption is not an aggressive act. The intestine does not seize nutrients—it allows them to pass through when conditions are right. This process depends on calm, coordinated movement and adequate time. When digestion is rushed or disrupted by stress, even the most nourishing material may pass through unused.

The nervous system plays a quiet but powerful role here. In states of urgency or anxiety, blood flow is diverted away from the digestive tract, slowing absorption. The body prioritizes survival over nourishment. What enters cannot be received.

Nourishment, it turns out, requires safety.

After the small intestine has extracted most usable material, the remaining contents move into the large intestine. Here, additional water is absorbed, and waste is compacted into solid form. This slow, deliberate process prepares the body for elimination. Eventually, waste reaches the rectum and exits the body, completing the digestive cycle.

But what happens when this process breaks down? Crohn's disease offers a real-life example of what a malfunctioning digestive system can look like. This autoimmune condition often unfolds in cycles—periods of painful "flares," when symptoms are active, followed by periods of remission.

In this state, discernment is lost. The digestive system, attempting to protect itself, begins rejecting nearly everything. Nourishment and waste are treated the same. But in guarding against perceived threats, it deprives the body of what it needs most—and in doing so, deepens the damage. Balance can only begin to return when the system is guided back toward intentional, selective function.

So what wisdom does the digestive system offer us?

It teaches us to be intentional about what we allow in—and equally intentional about what we release. Like the villi, we must remain selective, absorbing what nourishes us while refusing what causes harm. In life, nourishment comes in many forms: encouragement, meaningful work, supportive relationships, new skills, and experiences that foster confidence and growth. These are the building blocks that sustain us. Like a conversation with someone who listens without judgment—who can sit alongside you in the most difficult circumstances and offer support without even saying a word. These are the moments worthy of being absorbed; this is essential nutrition.

Just as importantly, we must learn to let go of what does not serve us. Maybe you have had conversations opposite of the one described above—ones that are long-winded and loud. Words come laced with urgency and criticism. How do you feel after these conversations?

Many of us cling to criticism, shame, pessimism, or resentment as though they are vital nutrients. In truth, they are waste–byproducts that must be processed and released. This does not mean that difficult emotions are inherently unhealthy. Sadness can cultivate empathy, and anger can motivate change when channeled constructively. But discernment remains key. Once the lesson has been extracted, the remainder must be let go.

Shame should never become part of your identity. Criticism should never define your worth. Like raw material in a forge, experiences—both good and painful—can be subjected to heat and reflection. What strengthens you may be shaped and built upon. What weakens you must be released. This is not cruelty—it is care.

When you choose what nourishes you and let go of what does not, you are not being selfish. You are being faithful to the wisdom of your body—a system designed not to hold everything, but to refine, sustain, and make room for life.

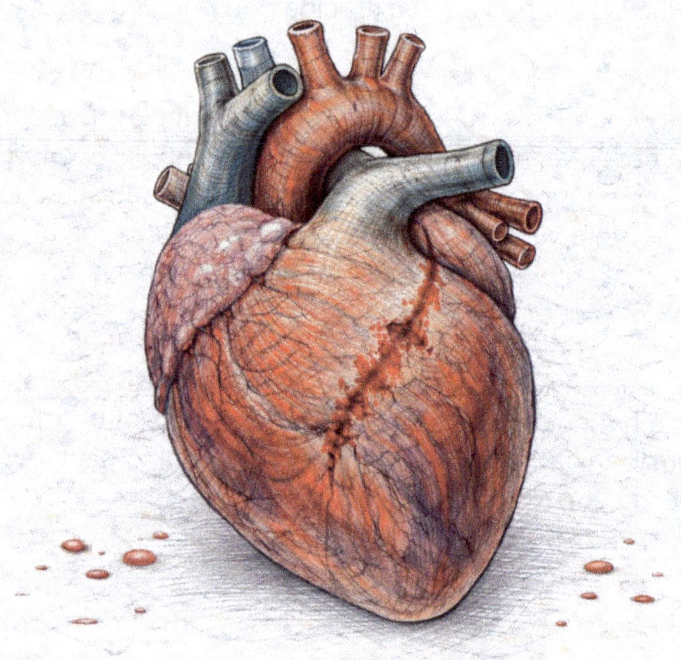

Heart:

Continuing to Beat After Pain

Heart: Continuing to Beat After Pain

We learn very early to associate the heart with life—and just as early, with pain. A steady heartbeat signals safety. An irregular one brings fear. We speak of broken hearts not because it is poetic, but because it is intuitive. Somewhere deep within us, we understand that the heart does more than move blood. It carries meaning.

Biologically, the heart is one of the smallest organs in the human body, weighing less than a pound. And yet, it labors without pause. It beats more than once per second, every second, for an entire lifetime. It responds to effort and to rest, to fear and to calm, to urgency and to safety. When demands rise, it accelerates. When conditions allow, it slows. It does not wait for instruction. It does not ask for recognition. When it functions well, we are scarcely aware of it. When it falters, everything else feels the strain.

Some forms of endurance are visible. Others are carried quietly.

This persistence does not develop over time—it is present from the very beginning. The heart is the first functional organ to form in the human body. Long before thought or memory, before language or intention, rhythm appears. Hearing that rhythm on a sonogram often brings parents to tears, not because of what it sounds like, but because of what it represents. Life has begun. And it intends to continue.

Structurally, the heart is divided into four chambers that work in precise coordination. Blood returning from the body enters the right side of the heart, travels to the lungs to receive oxygen, and then flows through the left side before being propelled outward again—delivering nourishment to every tissue. This cycle does not pause or reset. It continues, beat after beat, day after day, sustaining the body quietly and faithfully.

For such movement to occur without interruption, the heart relies on more than muscle alone. An internal electrical system governs each beat. The sinoatrial node—the heart's natural pacemaker—initiates the rhythm, sending signals through specialized pathways that ensure each contraction unfolds in proper sequence. When this timing is intact, the heart functions with remarkable efficiency. When it is disrupted, even a well-supplied heart can struggle, much like an engine misfiring despite a full tank.

Unlike machines, the heart does not simply wear down with use. When challenged appropriately, it often becomes stronger. With regular movement and sustained effort, new blood vessels can form, improving circulation and resilience. The heart remodels itself in response to demand. It is not fixed. It adapts.

But this capacity for adaptation does not make the heart indestructible.

When burdened by chronic stress, poor nourishment, inactivity, or sustained pressure, injury can occur. Chambers may enlarge and stiffen. Electrical rhythms may falter, leading to palpitations or arrhythmias. Plaque can accumulate in coronary arteries, restricting blood flow and increasing the risk of chest pain or heart attack. Damage may leave behind scar tissue or lingering inflammation. As the heart struggles, the effects ripple outward—fatigue deepens, breath shortens, thinking clouds, and even digestion may slow. The entire body carries the weight.

After such injury, it would seem reasonable to expect the heart to fail. To labor continuously for decades—especially while bearing the marks of damage—is no small task. And yet, even injured hearts continue. Blood flow may be redirected around blockages. New vessels can form. Rhythms adjust to compensate for tissue that no longer functions as it once did. Immune cells assist in clearing damage, shaping whether healing results in rigid scarring or more functional repair. While some injuries leave permanent marks, the heart does not abandon its purpose. It persists.

After injury, adaptation is not optimization—it is survival. A rerouted artery keeps blood flowing, but it does not mean the original path was meaningless. A shifted rhythm maintains function, but it carries the memory of what was lost.

This pattern extends beyond the physical body.

You may recognize this kind of persistence in yourself. Continuing to show up even when something inside you feels altered. Meeting obligations, maintaining routines, caring for others—while quietly aware that what once felt effortless now requires intention. From the outside, life looks unchanged. But internally, you are pacing yourself, measuring effort, conserving energy. You are still moving forward—just differently.

This endurance is quiet. It does not announce itself as suffering. And because it is so effective, it can go unnoticed—even by the one carrying it.

Humans often believe that heartbreak should end us. Loss reshapes us. Grief leaves marks that convince us we are broken beyond repair. In those moments, shutting down can feel safer than continuing—numbness easier than vulnerability, stillness less painful than hope. Many of us carry the belief, quietly and persistently, that pain has made us harder to love, that our scars are evidence of failure rather than proof of endurance.

Here is the wisdom the heart offers us: pain does not disqualify us from living.

Healing does not mean returning to who we were before. It means becoming someone new—someone shaped by experience, yet still capable of love, connection, and purpose. Like the heart, we are allowed to find new paths when old ones are blocked. Perhaps this is why the idea of "going back to who we were" feels impossible.

The heart does not return—it adapts.

And adaptation is not meant to shrink our lives. It is meant to preserve them. What begins as protection can, over time, become capacity again. Guarded souls can relax. Caution can coexist with courage. And what once felt risky may, in time, feel possible again.

The heart was never designed to heal in isolation.

Just as blood vessels, immune cells, and surrounding tissues support cardiac repair, we heal best in community. Others help bear the load. They soften the edges. They remind us that even after pain, rhythm can return.

The heart does not wait for perfect conditions to keep beating. It continues—imperfect, scarred, resilient. And in doing so, it teaches us this: survival is not the absence of injury. It is the courage to keep going anyway. And more than that—it is the quiet, persistent ability to live fully again.

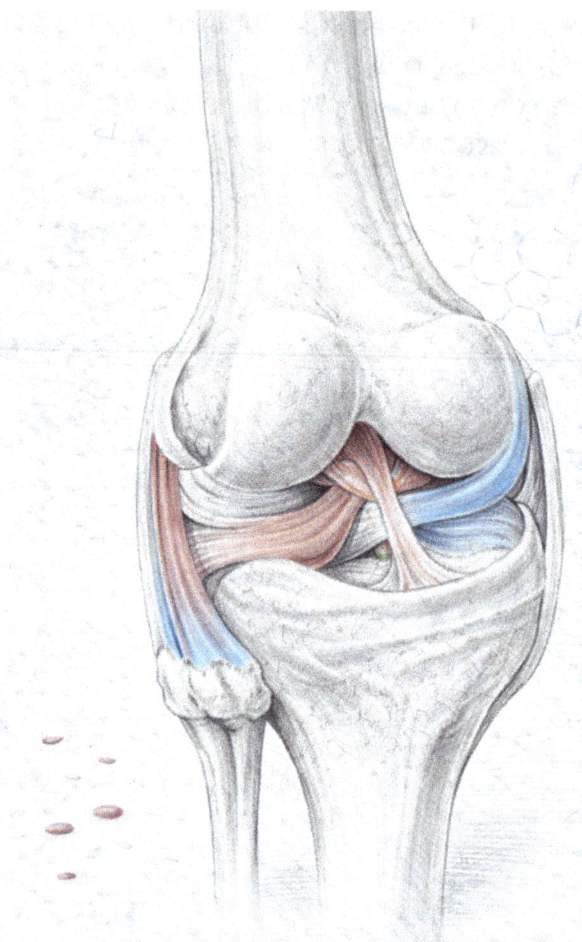

Bones and Joints:
Strength Requires Flexibility

Bones and Joints: Strength Requires Flexibility

When my son was very young, he went through a phase of fascination with construction vehicles—especially excavators. Any time we passed an excavation site while driving, he would strain against his seatbelt, craning his neck to catch even a glimpse of one through the window. His excitement was uncontainable. I've since learned that many parents share this experience; something about these massive machines captures the imagination of young children who are just beginning to make sense of the world. And perhaps they are right to marvel.

Excavators are remarkable not simply because of their size, but because of how they function. Thick steel beams provide structure and stability, while carefully placed joints and hydraulic systems allow for precise, adaptable movement. Strength alone would make the machine useless. Movement without structure would make it collapse. It is the relationship between the two that allows the excavator to do its work.

This same balance appears in the human body through the skeletal system.

The skeletal system is often regarded as one of the simpler body systems to understand. Compared to the microscopic complexity of other systems, it appears large, solid, almost mechanical. It consists of approximately 206 bones that form the structural framework of the body. But bones are not inert beams of steel. They are living tissue, constantly adapting to the demands placed upon them.

When subjected to repeated stress, bones respond by becoming denser and stronger, reinforcing themselves precisely where load is applied. This process allows the body to grow more capable over time, not by resisting force, but by responding to it.

Bones also provide the rigid framework against which muscles can pull, allowing force to be generated and movement to occur. Without bones, strength would have no anchor. And within their interior, bones contain marrow—reservoirs of stem cells that produce red blood cells, white blood cells, and platelets. In this way, the skeletal system not only supports the body, but sustains it.

The skeleton itself is divided into two main parts: the axial skeleton and the appendicular skeleton.

The axial skeleton consists of 80 bones that form the skull, vertebral column, and rib cage. These structures maintain our upright posture while protecting the most vital organs—the brain, spinal cord, heart, and lungs. Like the reinforced core of heavy machinery, the axial skeleton absorbs and redirects force away from what matters most, allowing us to move through the world without constant vulnerability.

The appendicular skeleton includes the remaining 126 bones and is primarily responsible for movement and exploration. The bones of the upper limbs allow reach, precision, and versatility. The pelvis bears and distributes the weight of the upper body, while the bones of the legs support balance, endurance, and forward motion. Together, these structures create a system that is both stable and mobile—capable of remarkable strength without sacrificing adaptability.

Yet bones alone would render us rigid and immobile.

Strength without movement is not useful. This is where joints become essential.

Joints are the connective structures that bind bones together and allow controlled movement. Cartilage cushions the ends of bones, reducing friction and absorbing shock. Synovial fluid lubricates joint surfaces, allowing smooth, low-resistance motion. Ligaments provide stability, holding bones together while permitting specific ranges of movement based on the joint's design.

Some joints, such as the knees and elbows, allow movement primarily in one direction, offering strength through limitation. Others, like the shoulders and hips, allow movement in multiple planes, providing flexibility and reach. But all joints have limits. When stressed beyond their natural range, injury can occur. Torn ligaments are reminders that flexibility without respect for structure can be just as damaging as rigidity.

The skeletal system teaches us something quietly profound: strength is not the absence of movement, but the ability to move without losing integrity.

Just as bones provide structure to the body, we rely on core values to provide structure in our lives. Truth, loyalty, love—these values form the framework upon which we build our choices and relationships. They support us, ground us, and give us something solid to lean on when life becomes heavy.

But values, like bones, are not meant to exist without joints.

You may have felt this tension yourself—when multiple paths seem equally valid, yet none feels completely right. Our values can pull against one another, caught in quiet conflict. We turn them over in our minds late at night, searching for the "correct" choice, and still wake feeling unsettled. This is the delicate work of balance: learning to stand firm without becoming rigid, and to bend without losing ourselves.

Truth may ask us to speak plainly, but relationships often require kindness and empathy as well. Loyalty can mean standing by someone's side—but it can also mean giving them space to grow. Love, perhaps most of all, changes shape over time. It adapts to growth, loss, and transformation. Love can bring joy and vitality. It can also bring sorrow and heartache. And sometimes, hardest of all, it asks us to let go of the people or roles we once held most tightly.

When values become completely rigid, they no longer support life—they restrict it. We become fixed, brittle, unable to adapt. Yet when values are forced to bend beyond recognition, we risk losing ourselves entirely. Just as joints have natural limits, so do our principles.

The wisdom of the skeleton lies in balance. Stand tall, but do not stand still. Bend when needed, but do not break. True strength is found not in unyielding rigidity, but in resilient structure—able to support, adapt, and endure. And just as the body requires both bones and joints, so do our hearts and minds: a foundation to rely on, and flexibility to navigate the unpredictable terrain of life.

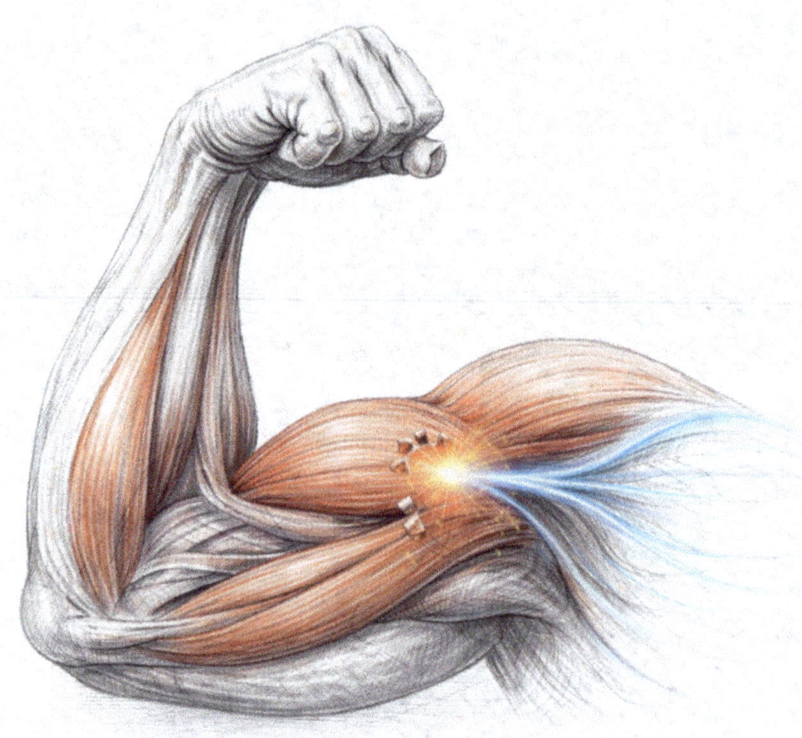

Muscles:

Growth Comes From Repair

Muscles: Growth Comes From Repair

Members of the muscular system could be described as the celebrities of the body. Like figures constantly in the public eye, muscles are praised when they are strong and visible—and scrutinized when they are not. Prominent skeletal muscles are often among the first things we notice about another's appearance, earning admiration or envy. At the same time, underdeveloped muscle can become a source of insecurity. Muscular appearance—or the lack of it—is a powerful motivator for exercise and self-improvement.

This emphasis is reflected in a single statistic: in the United States, people spend over thirty-five billion dollars each year on gym memberships alone. Yet these are only the muscles we can see. Beneath the surface, the muscular system performs work far more essential than appearance.

What we rarely see—and even more rarely honor—is the hidden work that makes strength possible after strain.

Muscles can be thought of as a busy construction site. Each muscle is composed of many workers, called fibers, whose job is to produce movement. Inside each fiber are smaller components—actin and myosin—that function like tools and tracks. Myosin pulls actin along these tracks in a coordinated sequence, much like workers tugging ropes to lift a heavy object. As actin and myosin slide past one another, the muscle shortens, producing contraction.

This process is directed by the nervous system. When an electrical signal arrives, it serves as a call to action. The fibers respond together, and movement occurs. This coordination can be seen simply by flexing a muscle, such as the biceps, and watching a long, flat structure gather into a dense peak.

Although all muscles rely on this basic mechanism, they differ significantly in form and function. Muscles fall into three main categories: cardiac, smooth, and skeletal.

Cardiac muscle, discussed in the heart chapter, is uniquely specialized. These muscle fibers initiate contraction through electrical signals generated by the sinoatrial node. To maintain precise timing, neighboring cells are connected by specialized junctions that allow signals to pass rapidly between them. This synchronization is essential. When it is disrupted, the consequences can be severe. Cardiac muscle functions involuntarily and tirelessly, sustaining life without conscious input for decades.

Smooth muscle is also involuntary and is found throughout the body. Governed by the autonomic nervous system, it adapts its contraction to meet local demands. In the digestive tract, smooth muscle moves food through the esophagus, stomach, and intestines. In blood vessels, it adjusts vessel diameter to regulate blood pressure. In the lungs, it controls airflow by narrowing or widening the airways. Smooth muscle also enables the urinary and reproductive systems to function. Unlike the shorter, more forceful contractions of skeletal muscle, smooth muscle sustains gentle contractions over long periods with remarkable efficiency.

Skeletal muscle is the type most associated with physical performance and strength training. These muscles enable movement, stabilize joints, and maintain posture. Unlike cardiac and smooth muscle, skeletal muscle is voluntary—we can contract and relax it at will. This control allows us to work, create, and pursue the activities that give life meaning. As explored in the skeletal system chapter, skeletal muscles function in partnership with bones to generate movement. Strength, however, is not determined by muscle size alone; it is also shaped by communication.

Muscle strength develops through two primary mechanisms.

The first is improved coordination between the nervous system and muscle fibers. With repeated use, muscles learn to contract more efficiently, reducing wasted effort and increasing endurance. This is similar to improving communication on a job site: better coordination leads to better outcomes without adding workers or tools.

When communication between nerves and muscles breaks down, strength is lost—not because the muscle disappears, but because the signal to use it no longer arrives. Conditions such as amyotrophic lateral sclerosis (ALS) illustrate this principle. As nerve cells lose their ability to communicate, muscles become weaker and less responsive. The structure remains, but direction is lost. This reveals an important truth: without clear communication, even the strongest systems cannot function.

The second mechanism of strength development is structural adaptation within the muscle fibers themselves. When muscles are repeatedly stressed, they undergo a process known as remodeling. Exercise creates microscopic damage—microtears—within muscle fibers. These small injuries activate the immune system, which clears damaged tissue and prepares the area for repair. Using nutrients from the diet, the body rebuilds the fibers with new proteins.

Importantly, the muscle is not merely restored to its previous state. The fibers become thicker, stronger, and more resilient. Like a construction site upgraded with better materials and refined processes, the muscle emerges better equipped to handle future demands. This repair continues for days after exercise ends—which is why rest is not a weakness, but an essential component of growth.

But this process depends on balance.

When stress overwhelms repair, harm replaces progress. Conditions such as rhabdomyolysis reveal what happens when muscle tissue breaks down faster than it can be rebuilt. In this state, inflammation accelerates damage rather than resolving it. Instead of becoming stronger, the tissue deteriorates. Stress without sufficient recovery does not produce resilience—it produces injury.

Without the capacity for repair, challenge would only wear us down. Injury would be purely destructive. Stress would offer no opportunity for growth—only depletion.

This pattern extends beyond the physical body.

Life introduces its own forms of microtrauma: long workdays, financial strain, difficult conversations, grief, and uncertainty. These experiences place demands on us much like exercise places demands on muscle. They carry the potential for growth—but only when strain is followed by rest and repair.

Renewal does not always arrive dramatically. Sometimes it looks like closing a laptop at the end of a long day and accepting that not everything can be solved tonight. It may mean recognizing that constant availability is not the same as commitment, or that rest is not a reward to be earned but a requirement for endurance. In these pauses, priorities can realign, and effort that once depleted us may begin to refine us instead.

Repair can also be quiet. It may appear as noticing a familiar reaction and choosing not to repeat it. A conversation revisited later. A boundary finally spoken. An apology offered or accepted. These moments do not erase the strain that came before them—but they allow experience to be transformed into understanding rather than resentment.

Challenge alone does not make us stronger. Without repair, stress only damages. Like muscles that cannot remodel, we risk becoming trapped in cycles of exhaustion and injury. Rest and reflection allow difficulty to serve a purpose. Self-compassion creates the conditions for resilience.

The body teaches us this: strength is built not through force alone, but through the careful balance of challenge and care. When we honor that balance, we complete the cycle—and grow into our full capacity.

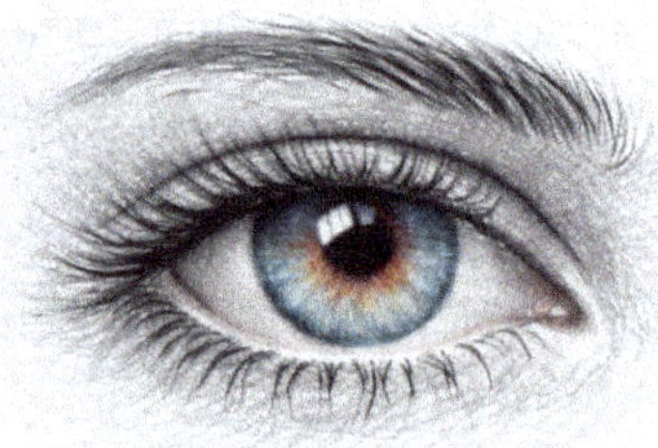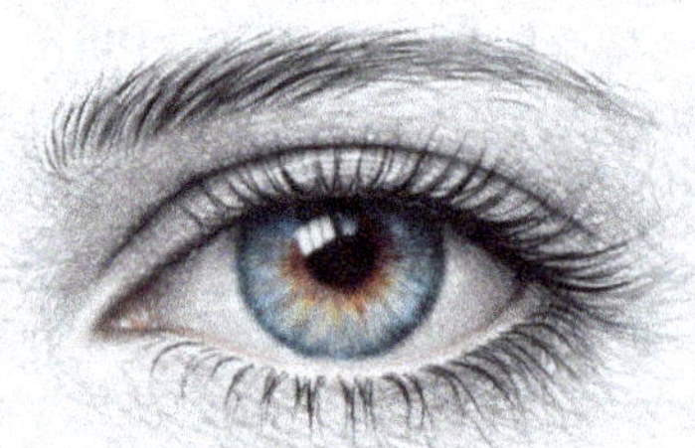

Eyes:

Rest Creates Clarity

Eyes: Rest Creates Clarity

While many of the systems we have discussed allow humans to interact directly with the world, the eyes serve a different purpose: they allow us to understand it from a distance. They are remarkable tools of perception, capable of gathering enormous amounts of information continuously throughout the day—like living cameras that rarely power down. Even more impressive is their ability to adapt effortlessly to changing conditions, whether in dim light, bright sun, or even underwater.

What the eyes reveal, over time, is that clarity is not achieved by looking harder—but by knowing when to rest.

Perhaps the most extraordinary function of the eyes, however, is not simply what they see—but what they anticipate. Vision allows us to predict motion before it fully unfolds. The simple act of hitting a baseball offers a powerful example. A professional player can perceive the pitch's speed and rotation, anticipate how the ball will move, predict where it will cross the plate, and decide whether to swing—all in less than half a second. This occurs seamlessly, as the nervous and muscular systems coordinate complex movements with precise timing. Before feeling frustrated with a player batting .150, it is worth pausing to appreciate the astonishing feat unfolding behind every swing.

It has often been said that the eyes are the windows to the soul. They are among the most expressive features of the human body, capable of conveying joy, fear, anger, or sorrow without a single word. But eyes do more than express emotion—they reveal interpretation. They show not only what we see, but how we see it. In this way, the eyes form a bridge between the external world and our internal one, shaping meaning as much as receiving information.

To better understand how the eyes accomplish this, it helps to compare them to a digital camera. Both systems are designed to sense and process light to produce an image. Light reflected off objects first passes through a protective filter—the cornea in the human eye—before traveling through a lens that focuses incoming rays. Cameras achieve focus by adjusting the position of glass elements inside the lens. As these elements move closer together or farther apart, the focal length changes, allowing objects at different distances to appear sharp.

The human eye performs this task automatically and continuously. Tiny ciliary muscles attached to the lens contract and relax, subtly changing its shape and adjusting focus in real time. You can experience this yourself. Choose an object close to you and focus on it. Without moving your eyes, notice the edges of your visual field—details there likely appear blurred. Now shift your focus to something farther away. Instantly, the distant object becomes clear while nearby objects blur. This transition happens effortlessly and almost instantaneously. Even with modern technology, few cameras can rival the eye's speed and precision.

When focusing intently, the eyes also perform subtle movements known as fixational movements. These tiny shifts ensure that visual cells are stimulated from slightly different angles. Without this constant variation, the cells would stop responding altogether. In other words, changing perspective is not optional—it is essential to maintaining vision itself.

Brightness, another crucial component of vision, is regulated by the iris. By adjusting the size of the pupil, the iris controls how much light enters the eye, much like a camera's aperture. At the back of a camera, a sensor absorbs light and converts it into electrical signals. In the human eye, this role is performed by the retina. But unlike a camera, the eye does not stop there. Electrical impulses generated by the retina travel through the optic nerve to the brain, where the image is interpreted, contextualized, and given meaning.

The speed of this process is staggering. The eye can transmit visual information to the brain at roughly ten million bits per second, and the brain can begin processing images in as little as thirteen milliseconds. This speed is critical. If vision or processing were delayed by even a single second, tasks like crossing a busy street would become dangerously impractical. Seeing is only one part of survival—the brain must immediately use visual information to guide movement through the nervous and muscular systems.

For all their sophistication, however, eyes are not built for endless strain. When focus is sustained too intensely for too long, the ciliary muscles fatigue. Like a camera running on a depleted battery, performance begins to suffer. Vision may blur or double. Concentration becomes difficult. Light, once essential, may cause discomfort. Reduced blinking can lead to dryness, redness, and irritation. Some people experience headaches or soreness around the eye sockets, making focus even more taxing. In these moments, clarity cannot be forced—it can only be restored through rest.

Our emotional lives often mirror this process with surprising accuracy.

When our perspective is healthy, we take in information fluidly, adjusting easily to different situations. We can see nuance. We extend empathy. Small frustrations are placed in context, and grace—for ourselves and others—comes more naturally.

But when emotional strain persists without rest, focus narrows. Perspective becomes rigid. We may begin to see only flaws in others and obstacles in our path. Empathy fades, not because we no longer care, but because we are exhausted. Problems feel heavier and more urgent than they truly are. We may complain or withdraw rather than process what we feel. If this experience sounds familiar, it is not a personal failure—it is a sign of fatigue.

Just as the eyes lose clarity when overworked, our emotional vision blurs when we are strained for too long. The remedy is the same: intentional rest.

Obsession and hyperfocus—whether on work, conflict, or worry—can distort perception. Just as the eye requires constant, subtle shifts to continue seeing, our emotional lives depend on gentle readjustment. Without it, clarity fades. Stepping away does not mean disengaging permanently; it means allowing space for perspective to reset. Often, understanding emerges not through effort, but through pause.

The eyes remind us that sometimes the best way to see clearly is to stop looking so hard.

Rest is not a luxury reserved for vacations or rare moments of escape. It is a daily requirement for clarity, discernment, and emotional health. When we honor the limits of our vision—both physical and emotional—we allow understanding to return. And with it, the ability to see the world, and ourselves, as they truly are.

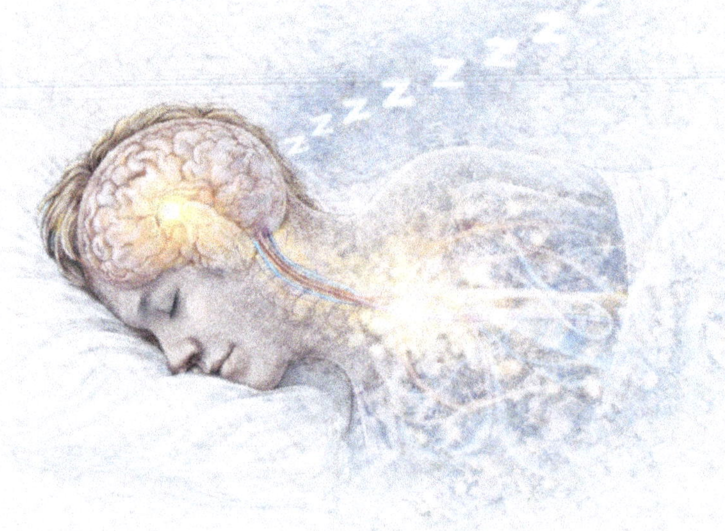

Sleep:

Healing Happens When We Stop

Sleep: Healing Happens When We Stop

At this point, we will step away from examining individual body systems to consider a process that affects them all: sleep. Just as the eyes must occasionally rest to restore clarity, this chapter is meant to serve a similar purpose as we enter the second half of this book—a pause that allows deeper repair and renewed perspective. Thank you for continuing on this journey.

Sometimes the most meaningful change does not come from doing more—but from allowing ourselves to stop.

"I'll sleep when I'm dead."

The phrase is familiar, almost celebrated. It reflects a cultural attitude that treats sleep as optional—an inconvenience to be minimized in favor of productivity. But what does science say? More importantly, what does your body say after sleep has been sacrificed for too long? And are we listening?

Sleep is not a passive state. It is an active, highly organized process essential to survival.

Scientifically, sleep is divided into two primary categories: non–rapid eye movement (NREM) sleep and rapid eye movement (REM) sleep. NREM sleep itself is divided into three distinct stages, each offering unique benefits.

NREM Stage 1 (N1) marks the transition from wakefulness to sleep. This stage lasts five to ten minutes and is characterized by light sleep, slowed brain activity, and reduced muscle tone. Awakening is easy.

NREM Stage 2 (N2) follows, lasting roughly twenty to thirty minutes per cycle. Heart rate and body temperature begin to drop, and brain activity slows further as the body settles into true sleep.

NREM Stage 3 (N3)—often called deep or slow-wave sleep—lasts approximately twenty to forty minutes per cycle. This is the deepest stage of sleep and the most difficult to awaken from. While every stage serves a purpose, N3 is widely regarded as the most critical for physical recovery, tissue repair, and systemic restoration.

The final stage is REM sleep, occurring about ninety minutes after falling asleep and lasting ten to twenty minutes per cycle. During REM sleep, brain activity increases, rapid eye movements occur, and vivid dreaming takes place. Many awakenings happen during or shortly after this stage.

A complete sleep cycle progresses as follows:

N1 → N2 → N3 → N2 → REM

Over the course of a healthy night, this cycle typically repeats four to six times. Sleep needs vary by life stage—newborns may require up to seventeen hours per day, while most adults function best with approximately eight.

Sleep is only fully restorative when these cycles are allowed to unfold uninterrupted. Fragmented sleep—frequent awakenings, shortened nights, or inconsistent schedules—prevents the body from completing its work. Repair begins but remains unfinished, night after night. The result is not immediate collapse, but gradual deficit: healing deferred, clarity dulled, resilience quietly eroded.

Although consciousness fades during sleep, internal work accelerates.

Growth hormone, for example, is released primarily during N3 deep sleep. While often associated with childhood growth, it remains essential throughout adulthood—supporting muscle repair, fat metabolism, bone density, and tissue regeneration across every system. Muscles rebuild. Bones strengthen. Even the small muscles of the eyes recover their ability to focus. Appetite-regulating hormones recalibrate, overstimulated nerves quiet, and immune signaling molecules are replenished.

The brain is equally active. The hypothalamus—small but powerful—coordinates hormone release, regulates body temperature, and guides transitions between sleep stages. During sleep, toxins that accumulate during wakefulness are cleared from the brain. Energy reserves are restored. Memories are replayed, organized, and integrated, strengthening recall and improving problem-solving.

Emotional experiences are also processed during sleep. Feelings that were too heavy, confusing, or overwhelming during the day are softened and integrated at night. This helps explain why sleep deprivation is so closely linked to anxiety, depression, and emotional reactivity—and why the advice to "sleep on it" so often proves wise. Time and rest succeed where effort alone cannot.

This subject carries personal significance for me.

For five years, I worked overnight shifts at a small community hospital. The transition from a traditional schedule to nocturnal work was not kind. Within weeks, I experienced body aches, headaches, severe mood changes, anxiety, and depression. These symptoms made sleep increasingly difficult, creating a cycle that fed itself.

The arrangement was justified—financial security, fewer childcare hours away from my young son. On paper, it made sense. In reality, I was slowly disappearing.

I became a shell of myself without realizing it. Only after returning to a day shift did I recognize how much vitality, patience, and joy had been lost. If you find yourself in a similar position, please hear this: I want better for you. While a small number of people may tolerate overnight work well, most cannot sustain it without cost. Sleep cannot be postponed and repaid later. It is a daily biological requirement.

Too often, we treat wakefulness as something to be extended indefinitely—borrowing energy from tomorrow to survive today. Caffeine and stimulation prop us up just long enough to feel functional, even sharp. But the debt accumulates quietly. Eventually, the body will demand repayment, and it will do so on its own terms.

Many cultures—particularly American culture—equate rest with weakness. Productivity is praised; stillness is suspect. When demands increase, we create no space. When finances strain, we add work. When exhaustion sets in, sleep is often the first thing sacrificed.

This is not strength. It is erosion.

The body tells a different story. Rest is not earned; it is essential. Stopping is not failure—it is an active process of renewal. Healing requires periods of reduced input, allowing waste to be cleared and repair to occur. In a world of constant stimulation, sleep remains one of the few spaces where consumption ceases and restoration begins.

We are not machines. We are living systems. And living systems require regular, intentional pauses to function with clarity, resilience, and grace.

Healing happens when we stop.

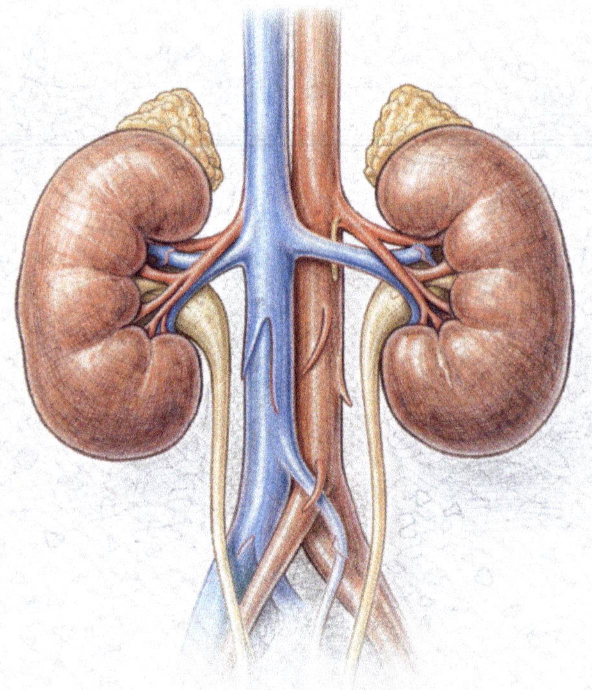

Kidneys:

Quiet, Unseen Work

Kidneys: Quiet, Unseen Work

Have you ever been invited to a pool party? Perhaps you even own a pool yourself. Some of my favorite childhood memories were made in and around swimming pools—cannonball contests, daring leaps from diving boards, the thrill of trying to make an athletic catch just before crashing into the water below. Few environments allow children to take such joyful risks. As adults, pool life may look different: floating lazily with a drink in hand, or lounging nearby while soaking in the warmth of the sun. However we experience them, pools often represent leisure, freedom, and rest.

But anyone who owns a pool knows that this enjoyment depends entirely on something less glamorous: maintenance. Crystal-clear water does not happen by chance. Behind the scenes, filtration systems run continuously, and chemical balance must be carefully maintained. Neglect turns a beautiful oasis into a stagnant eyesore.

Much of what keeps us well—physically and emotionally—depends on work that is never seen, but felt when it is missing.

In the body, this responsibility belongs to the kidneys.

Kidneys rarely draw attention when they are functioning well. Like pool filters, they work silently and continuously, often unnoticed. But when filtration falters, the consequences spread quickly and affect nearly every system.

The kidneys are two small, bean-shaped organs located just below the rib cage, one on each side of the spine. Each weighs only ten to twelve ounces, yet they sit strategically between the body's largest blood vessels—the aorta and the vena cava—allowing constant access to blood flow. Despite their size, the kidneys receive roughly twenty-five percent of the heart's total output. Their importance cannot be overstated.

Each kidney is composed of two primary regions. The outer layer, the renal cortex, is where filtration and decision-making occur. Blood enters microscopic filtering units, and enormous volumes of fluid are processed—nearly thirty times the body's total blood volume each day. Like a pool filter catching debris, the cortex removes waste products and excess substances from circulation.

But filtration alone is not enough. What follows is discernment.

The filtered fluid travels through an intricate network of tubules where reabsorption takes place. Water, glucose, amino acids, proteins, and electrolytes are selectively reclaimed and returned to the bloodstream. This process preserves what the body needs while allowing the rest to be released. Here, the kidneys regulate pH—maintaining a narrow balance between acidity and alkalinity that is essential for survival. Even slight deviations can disrupt muscle function, nerve signaling, and metabolism. Pool owners may recall the frustration of correcting water chemistry by hand; the kidneys perform this balancing act continuously and without effort.

The remaining filtrate then enters the renal medulla, the inner portion of the kidney. Here, the focus shifts toward concentration and release. Water is reclaimed with precision, while waste becomes increasingly concentrated. By the end of this process, waste is directed into the ureters and transported to the bladder for elimination.

Beyond filtration, the kidneys also serve as hormonal regulators. When oxygen levels drop, they release erythropoietin, stimulating the bone marrow to produce new red blood cells. They activate calcitriol, enabling calcium absorption essential for bone strength and cellular function. And through the release of renin, they help govern long-term blood pressure control. While the heart and blood vessels respond quickly to short-term demands, the kidneys provide stability over time.

For such small organs, the kidneys carry an extraordinary burden. Yet they perform this work with quiet persistence—a relentless commitment to balance and refinement.

What happens when that work is disrupted?

Because the kidneys are deeply integrated with every other system, injury or disease affecting them is among the most dangerous conditions the body can endure. Acute kidney injury is a sudden loss of function that can occur over days, often triggered by dehydration, heart failure, severe illness, or certain medications. Like pool water clouded after a storm, balance is lost quickly. Waste accumulates, pH shifts, muscles may spasm uncontrollably, and electrolyte disturbances can trigger dangerous heart rhythms. In severe cases, dialysis—external filtration of the blood—may be required. When addressed promptly, recovery can be rapid.

Chronic kidney disease, however, unfolds slowly—over months or years—most often due to diabetes or long-standing high blood pressure. The damage accumulates quietly. Early symptoms are minimal. Subtle losses occur as nutrients that should be reabsorbed are instead discarded. Over time, the consequences surface: uncontrolled blood pressure, swelling, anemia, fatigue, and eventual kidney failure requiring lifelong dialysis or transplantation. Even then, full restoration is rare. Damage that accrues silently over years cannot be undone easily.

This is why the kidneys' invisible labor must be protected.

Much of our emotional health depends on similar quiet work. It rarely draws attention. It earns no applause. No one congratulates you for sitting with grief, or for choosing not to respond in anger, or for recognizing resentment before it hardens into identity. And yet, this unseen labor is essential. Processing feelings, setting internal boundaries, releasing bitterness—these are the emotional equivalents of filtration and balance.

Many of us carry complicated relationships with our emotions. We may grow frustrated with ourselves for feeling angry or sad, telling ourselves to move on as though emotions were obstacles rather than information. Some come to see sorrow or despair as personal weakness—evidence that we are not resilient enough or grateful enough. Society reinforces this belief by sorting emotions into categories: joy and gratitude labeled "positive," fear, regret, or grief labeled "negative."

This framing does harm. Emotions are signals, not verdicts. We do not need to judge ourselves for feeling them. We are invited to experience them fully and without guilt—to give them space rather than rushing to silence them. Every emotion carries information worth hearing. Even painful feelings can teach us what we value, what we fear, and what we need.

When the time comes to respond, we are not asked to react impulsively or suppress ourselves into numbness. We are asked to respond with intention and care. In doing so, we acknowledge our emotions without allowing them to rule us. We create balance. We restore flow.

Life inevitably causes internal damage. An unexpected tragedy can leave us disoriented and powerless. Anger, fear, and sadness may surge all at once—and that response is not a failure. It is human. When we meet these emotions quickly and intentionally, we honor them while limiting the harm they can cause.

But when hardship remains unaddressed—when emotions are ignored, dismissed, or buried—they begin to accumulate. Slowly and quietly, they erode our well-being. From the outside, we may appear fine. Functional. Capable. But beneath the surface, imbalance grows. Fatigue deepens. Joy dulls. Connection weakens. A life spent clinging to bitterness does not collapse all at once—it becomes heavy, rigid, and numb.

The body teaches us that healing comes from deliberate filtering. From reabsorption and release. From a return to balance. The work is slow, patient, and often invisible—but it is the work that preserves life. And though it may never be noticed by anyone else, it is noticed by you. Quietly, steadily, it restores clarity.

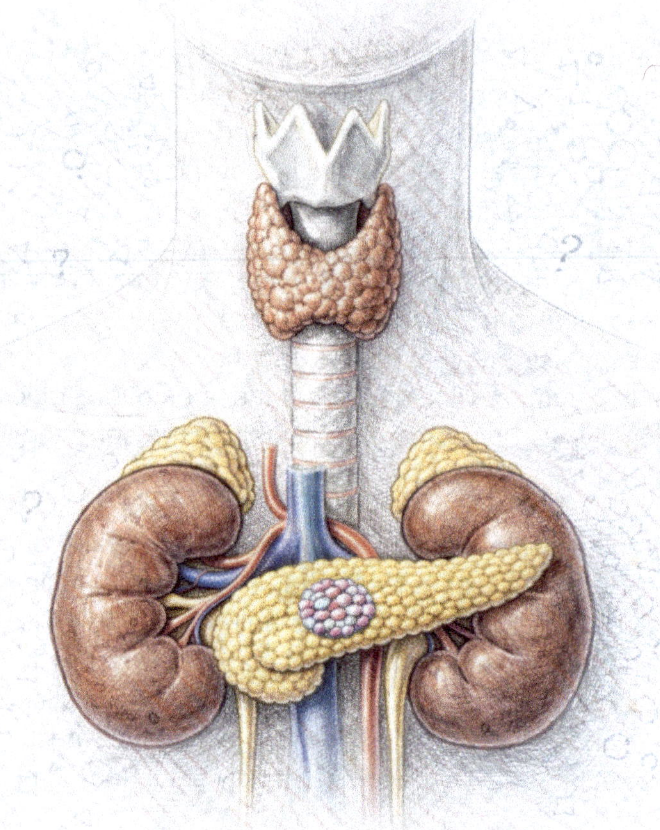

Endocrine System:

Small Imbalances Have Big Effects

Endocrine System: Small Imbalances Have Big Effects

Imagine a suspended balance system—a delicate mobile hanging from the ceiling. Lightweight arms extend outward, each carrying a carefully weighted element. At first glance, it appears still. But it is never truly at rest. A change in weight anywhere forces the entire structure to reorganize. The smallest nudge to a single piece sends all the others shifting, adjusting, seeking equilibrium once again. This image offers a fitting way to understand the endocrine system.

Over time, we discover that the most destabilizing forces in life are rarely dramatic—they are small imbalances sustained without attention.

Inside each human body exists an intricate network of chemical messengers—a web of cause and effect that quietly governs nearly every function. These messengers, known as hormones, influence metabolism, growth, mood, sleep, reproduction, and far more. No hormone acts in isolation. The endocrine system is composed of multiple glands releasing hormones into circulation, each signal shaping and reshaping the body's internal environment. Many of the systems we have already explored depend on this network, responding constantly to its cues. Harmony is not optional; it is the requirement.

Hormonal regulation relies on feedback loops—mechanisms that function much like a home's temperature control system. When a room becomes too warm or too cold, a thermostat senses the deviation and signals the appropriate system to activate. Once balance is restored, the signal quiets, and the system stands down. One device may govern opposing functions—heating and cooling—responding appropriately depending on need. This closed loop allows stability without excess.

The endocrine system operates in much the same way.

A clear example is the pancreas, which plays a central role in regulating blood glucose. After a meal, nutrients flood the bloodstream. Glucose becomes abundant, ready to be used for energy or stored for later. The pancreas senses this rise and releases insulin. Insulin signals cells throughout the body to absorb glucose and directs the liver to store excess energy as glycogen or fat. Much like saving leftovers after dinner, the body preserves resources for times when intake is limited. As glucose leaves the bloodstream and enters cells, blood sugar returns to its optimal range—and insulin secretion subsides.

When food intake is delayed or skipped, the opposite signal is required. As blood sugar drops, the pancreas releases glucagon. This hormone instructs the liver to break down stored glycogen and fat, converting them back into usable glucose. During prolonged fasting, glucagon also promotes the creation of new glucose from other sources, such as protein. Once nourishment is restored, glucagon is no longer needed and quietly recedes.

The relationship between insulin and glucagon illustrates the central principle of endocrine regulation: balance maintained through opposition. Neither hormone dominates. Each responds precisely, activating when needed and standing down when its role is complete.

Many readers are familiar with these hormones because disruptions in this system give rise to diabetes mellitus. When balance is lost, blood sugar swings dramatically. In type 1 diabetes, insulin production fails. Glucose enters the bloodstream but remains inaccessible to cells, circulating far longer than intended and damaging tissues in its wake. In type 2 diabetes, insulin is present—often in abundance—but cells become resistant to its message. The signal is broadcast repeatedly, yet no longer received.

Over time, this imbalance takes a toll. Small blood vessels are damaged, impairing vision and kidney function. Nerves are injured, causing pain, tingling, or numbness. Wounds heal poorly. Cardiovascular risk rises. These consequences rarely arrive suddenly. They accumulate quietly, one imbalance reinforcing another, until the body's ability to compensate is exhausted. Tiny hormonal shifts, sustained over time, can reshape an entire life.

Despite this fragility, some have attempted to harness hormones for performance rather than balance. In competitive sports, artificial amplification of hormonal signals has promised strength, endurance, or recovery beyond natural limits. Athletes such as Lance Armstrong and the players implicated by the Mitchell Report learned a difficult lesson: when one signal is forced to dominate, the system itself collapses. Performance gained at the expense of balance is never sustainable. Health, trust, and future potential are often the cost.

Hormones teach us something deeper than physiology. They reveal how balance—not dominance—allows complexity to function.

Each of us carries multiple roles: parent, partner, professional, friend, student, caregiver, dreamer. These roles generate emotions that rise and fall constantly. How do we hold all of it?

Consider comfort. There is something deeply satisfying about rest—being home on a familiar couch, wrapped in a warm blanket, surrounded by ease. Perhaps your favorite snack is within reach while a familiar show plays softly in the background. Many of us could stay there indefinitely. But when comfort becomes our only pursuit, growth stalls. Health suffers. Meaning fades.

Now consider the opposite extreme: relentless motion. Constant striving. Exercise without rest. Achievement without pause. Momentum becomes identity. Relationships thin. Joy loses depth. Accomplishment grows hollow when there is no one left to share it with. I have lived seasons on both ends of this spectrum, and neither felt complete.

External balance is essential. Work must make room for rest. Effort must allow recovery. Neither indulgence nor deprivation leads to wholeness.

The same is true internally.

One of the most poignant illustrations of this truth appears in the film *Inside Out*, where a young girl learns that prioritizing joy at the expense of all other emotions fractures her inner world. Sadness, anger, and fear are not enemies. Like hormones, emotions are not meant to dominate—they are meant to inform. Each carries a message. Each has a role.

Joy enriches life, but sorrow teaches empathy. Anger can spark change. Fear can protect. Emotional balance often means holding opposing feelings at once—gratitude and grief after a loss, pride and longing at a graduation, hope and uncertainty when beginning something new. These combinations are not contradictions; they are evidence of depth.

Like the mobile at the beginning of this chapter, our lives function best not when one element outweighs all others, but when every signal is acknowledged and allowed to play its part. Small imbalances matter. But so does our remarkable capacity to adjust—to listen, to respond, and to return, again and again, to equilibrium.

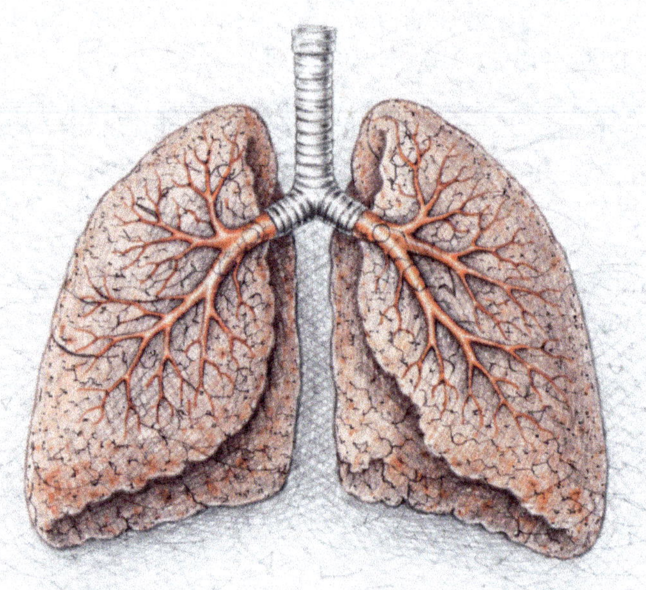

Lungs:

Courage to Trust

Lungs: Courage to Trust

In the quiet internal world of the womb, nature is a patient architect—yet it saves the most vital threshold for last. The lungs are the final organs to reach maturity, as if the body understands that the transition from being held to being whole is the most delicate task of all. For parents of a premature infant, this biological delay is not a mere fact of development but an agonizing introduction to the fragility of life—a season of waiting where every rise and fall of a tiny chest becomes a prayer for independence.

This struggle reveals a truth we often forget as we grow: that our very survival depends on a constant, rhythmic exchange. To breathe is to enter into a contract of radical trust—a commitment to draw in the world around us and, just as importantly, the courage to let it go.

In humans, oxygen is essential for energy production. We rely on this corrosive and potentially dangerous gas every moment, craving it with every breath. The respiratory process begins with inhalation, when air is drawn into the lungs. The diaphragm, a large muscle beneath the lungs, contracts and moves downward, creating space within the chest. At the same time, the muscles between the ribs contract, expanding the rib cage and enlarging the chest cavity even further.

This expansion creates negative pressure inside the lungs, and air rushes in through the nose and mouth to restore balance.

Contrary to popular belief, breathing is not something we accomplish through effort alone—it is an agreement with the laws of nature. We are responsible only for making space. Nature does the rest.

Inhaled air travels down the trachea, or windpipe, and into the lungs as they expand. Within each lung are millions of tiny air sacs called alveoli, each surrounded by a dense network of capillaries. Here, the most intimate exchange occurs. Oxygen passes through the thin walls of the alveoli and into the bloodstream, where it is carried back to the heart and distributed throughout the body, delivering energy and sustaining life. At the same time, carbon dioxide—a waste product of metabolism—moves out of the blood and into the alveoli to be exhaled.

Once this exchange is complete, the diaphragm relaxes and moves upward. The rib cage returns to its resting position. Pressure within the chest increases, and the lungs recoil, expelling carbon dioxide-rich air and preparing the body for the next breath. The only way to take a new life-giving breath is to empty ourselves of the old one.

If this rhythm is disrupted for even a few minutes, the consequences can be terrifying. Obstructive lung diseases offer a stark reminder of how fragile this balance is. Asthma, one such condition, is often triggered by allergens carried in inhaled air. When these particles are detected, the body's defenses activate immediately. The tissues lining the airways become inflamed, smooth muscles tighten, and thick mucus is secreted to trap potential threats.

These responses are not irrational. They are designed to protect. And they are remarkably effective at capturing invaders.

But they also restrict the airflow required to survive. Effortless breathing quickly transforms into wheezing, coughing, and panic as the diaphragm and surrounding muscles strain desperately to move air through narrowing passages.

Exhalation becomes just as difficult as inhalation. Without a full release, carbon dioxide builds up within the lungs, crowding out oxygen and occupying precious space. Dizziness, confusion, shortness of breath, and even seizures may follow as the body struggles under the weight of its own defenses. If allowed to continue, this internal battle can become life-threatening. And even after an episode resolves, fear often lingers—limiting participation in activities once enjoyed, shrinking life to avoid the possibility of another attack.

What makes this response so tragic is that it begins as an attempt to stay safe. The body is not acting irrationally—it is responding to remembered danger. But when protection becomes reflexive rather than responsive, it begins to threaten the very life it seeks to preserve.

Yet for all our fragility, humans have no way to stockpile breath—no way to hoard oxygen for seasons of hardship. Aggressive responses that shut out the external world also sever our access to life-giving exchange. Whether the threat is a harmless allergen or a dangerous pathogen, complete shutdown would cause more harm than good. Defense in excess becomes its own form of destruction.

The only way to breathe fully again is to decompress the body's overreaction—to return to relaxed, rhythmic exchange. This requires trust: trust in the body's ability to regulate, trust in nature's laws, and trust that safety does not come from control alone. The lungs demand presence. Every breath is an act of intimate reliance, anchored firmly in the present moment.

This pattern of trust extends far beyond the physical body.

Pain has a quiet way of shrinking our world. Past relationships may fill us with insecurity, and trauma may crowd us with doubt. Perhaps you have felt it in your chest—the tightening before a conversation, the instinct to withdraw just as connection feels possible. Or the quiet internal negotiations—the ways we explain, soften, or look away from discomfort in an effort to protect ourselves. You may tell yourself that you are better off alone, shielded from feeling like a burden, shielded from being hurt again.

But protection that never loosens eventually becomes confinement. What begins as self-preservation slowly limits our capacity to receive what we need most. Like holding the breath for too long, withdrawal creates the illusion of control while quietly depriving us of oxygen. Release, then, is not carelessness—it is courage. It is the decision to exhale despite uncertainty, trusting not that harm will never come, but that you can survive it if it does.

Like the hormones of the endocrine system, humans are not designed to function in isolation. Community is as essential to us as the air we breathe. Our differing perspectives challenge us to grow. We compensate for one another's blind spots. Deep relationships provide meaning, support, and a sense of belonging that cannot be replicated alone.

To live fully, we must make space. We must release what no longer serves us so that something new can enter. And that requires trust—not only in others, but within ourselves.

You may wonder what happens when new relationships awaken old pain. This is a valid fear. New connections will bring new challenges, and some will hurt. But trust is not the absence of risk—it is confidence in your ability to respond. When familiar pain surfaces, the instinct to shut down must be gently challenged, not obeyed. Internal boundaries—formed through reflection and experience—allow us to engage without losing ourselves.

Like the lungs, we are called to live in the present moment. To inhale fully. To exhale completely. To trust that we are capable of adapting and recovering. You do not need to be afraid of letting others in. Like your lungs, you were built not merely to survive—but to trust the rhythm of exchange that makes life possible.

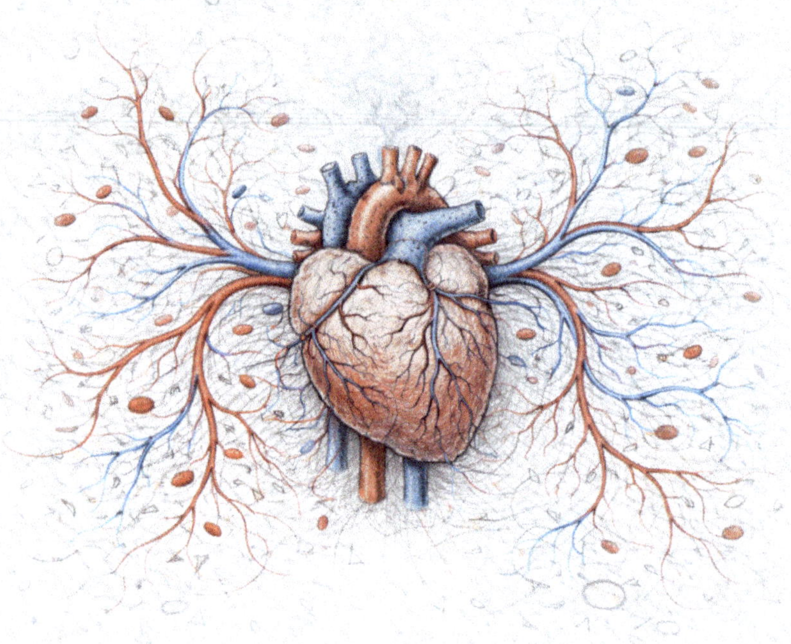

Circulatory System:
Let Connection Flow

Circulatory System: Let Connection Flow

The circulatory system is one we have already touched upon in several other chapters. And for good reason: the blood vessels that make up this system are intimately woven into every other aspect of the body. Like a network of highways and local roads, blood vessels form the transport framework for the body's resources. This work may not be glamorous or flashy, but it is essential for connection, function, and support.

Blood may look like a simple red fluid, but it is a living mixture—cells, proteins, nutrients, and signals moving together as one. Red blood cells carry oxygen, bringing life and energy everywhere they go, and they also pick up carbon dioxide waste to bring back to the lungs for removal. White blood cells patrol for threats, sensing and neutralizing danger when it arises. Hormones, clotting proteins, glucose, amino acids—these and more use the bloodstream as a shared transit system. And plasma, though easy to overlook, is the medium that lets everything move. Without it, even the most capable cells cannot flow to where they are needed.

So we know that the blood holds vital constituents and moves through the circulatory system. But how? What does that movement look like? To begin, let's return to an old friend: the heart. As we explored previously, the heart is the engine that drives circulation. Its rhythmic and reliable pulse marks both the launch and the return of the bloodstream.

The circulatory system relies on three major types of vessels: arteries, capillaries, and veins. Arteries carry blood away from the heart—often oxygen-rich, though not always. The largest artery in the body, the aorta, begins just above the heart and has thick, resilient walls capable of carrying trillions of blood cells at any given moment. From there, arteries branch outward across the body, dividing again and again, becoming smaller as they reach the furthest places.

Arteries continue to narrow until they become capillaries, the tiniest blood vessels. Their walls are only one cell thick, and they are so small that red blood cells must slow down and travel single file. But do not let their size fool you—this is where the most intimate exchange happens between blood and tissue. This combination of vulnerability and slow intention is required for nourishment to enter and for harmful waste to be removed. And perhaps this is worth noticing: the body delivers its most essential support not through force, but through closeness—by slowing down enough for transfer to occur. Once capillaries have delivered their cargo, they begin to merge and pool their now-depleted blood into larger vessels once more.

Veins complete the work capillaries begin. They carry unoxygenated blood and waste back toward the heart and lungs. Carrying waste may not sound glorious, but it is critical to the health of the whole body. Energy and life are not enough on their own; what is depleted must be carried away so toxicity does not build. As veins approach the heart, many merge into the vena cava—the largest veins in the body, delivering directly into the heart. From there, blood is pumped to the lungs, where it releases carbon dioxide and receives fresh oxygen, and the cycle begins again.

Blood vessels, however, are not immune to pathology. High blood pressure can place constant, excess force on the walls of arteries, narrowing them and making them less elastic over time. This strain can reach a breaking point when an artery wall weakens, bulges, and ruptures—an aneurysm capable of life-threatening bleeding. Plaque from excess cholesterol may also accumulate gradually within artery walls, causing vessels to harden and narrow. Depending on location, reduced blood flow can lead to chest pain, shortness of breath, kidney damage, and more.

These conditions are often called "silent killers" because the true extent of their damage can remain unseen until it is severe. The body adapts. It compensates. It reroutes. It keeps moving—until it can't.

One of the most perilous consequences of vascular damage is a blood clot: a total blockage of flow that can occur anywhere in the body. The most dangerous clots affect the heart, lungs, and brain. Clots in the coronary arteries deprive the heart of oxygen, causing what most know as a heart attack. A blockage in the lungs is a pulmonary embolism. Both may begin with chest pain, shortness of breath, dizziness, and fear—and both can become life-threatening with terrifying speed. Even with recovery, lasting effects can remain: abnormal heart rhythms, scarred tissue, diminished function.

Perhaps most urgent of all is a clot in the brain—a stroke. The brain is especially sensitive to changes in blood flow and oxygen. If it is deprived for even a few minutes, brain cells begin to die. Long-term effects can include paralysis, speech difficulties, memory impairment, and profound changes to identity and ability. Connection must be maintained constantly within the body, extending to every part. When circulation is cut off, tissue dies—and the whole organism suffers.

Just as the body knows the importance of connection, our souls do too.

A relationship—whether it is a lifelong friendship, a familial bond, or a romantic partnership—is far more than a simple contract between two people; it is a living, breathing organism. While we often focus on the external milestones of our lives, the true vitality of any bond lies in its internal circulatory system of connection. This system does not just transport words; it carries the vital nutrients of shared presence, physical touch, emotional safety, and mutual support. Just as blood must reach the furthest extremities of the body to prevent atrophy, connection must move into every corner of a relationship to keep it from withering. When we are truly connected, we live in a state of constant, rhythmic exchange—giving and receiving the invisible resources that sustain our spirits. To neglect that exchange is to risk more than misunderstanding; it is to allow the relationship to slowly starve. Ultimately, connection is the pulse of our shared humanity—the essential current that ensures no part of us has to survive alone.

Relationships are not built in a single moment; a single instant of connection cannot sustain us forever. True connection between people requires the steady pulse of consistency. Like blood, partnership is composed of many different parts. The oxygen of shared laughter and new experiences keeps relationships energized. Healthy boundaries protect us from infections such as jealousy or doubt. And empathy acts like plasma—reducing friction so feelings can move freely rather than clotting in silence.

As blood vessels teach us, this flow cannot exist in only one direction. Well-being requires both giving and receiving. Support must flow outward through acts of service, physical affection, and the simple act of making space. These actions are life-giving. Perhaps even more difficult is allowing that same flow to return to you—allowing yourself to be seen, helped, and carried. Some of us can offer help easily and feel exposed the moment we need it. But receiving does not make you weak; it allows others to fulfill their role in the system and complete the circuit of trust.

Connection does not always look like grand gestures or long conversations. Most often, the real life of relationships grows in the smallest moments—the places where we are forced to slow down and exchange. These are the moments when we sit in comfortable silence, heads on shoulders while fingers are intertwined. Small gestures that anticipate each other's needs. Kind words and reassurance offered without being asked. This is where the true nourishment happens: quiet transfers of energy that occur simply by being in one another's presence.

Any obstacle that threatens to interrupt this flow can cause damage. Prolonged seasons of stress put excessive force on the framework of even the strongest relationship. When connection is defined by chronic tension, frequent criticism, or unresolved conflict, the relationship loses its ability to be flexible, patient, and resilient in the face of life's challenges. If small grievances are allowed to accumulate over time, the path for honest communication becomes narrow and strained.

A relationship can look intact from the outside—shared schedules, shared space, shared history—while the flow inside has quietly slowed. Conversations become transactional. Touch becomes infrequent. Needs go unmet not from malice, but from disconnection. Like tissue deprived of blood, parts of the relationship grow numb long before anyone names it. And a complete shutdown of communication can threaten catastrophic damage to everyone involved, leaving long-term ramifications in its wake. We ought not to shy away from the difficult conversations that can clear these blockages; to do so is to risk everything.

We are circulatory creatures by design. Just as every part of the body depends on the blood delivered through its vessels, every part of our souls yearns for true kinship: to be known and to know others, to teach and to learn, to love and to be loved. We are not meant to be separate systems sealed off from one another. Living fully requires participation in the constant, rhythmic exchange of connection—because it is the only thing that can bring life to every part of us.

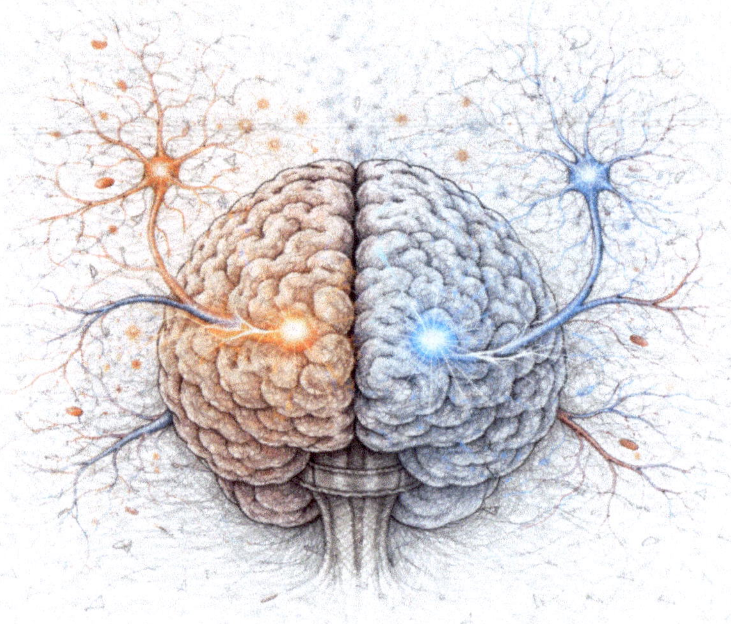

Brain:

Change Is Always Possible

Brain: Change Is Always Possible

There is a comforting but dangerous lie we often tell ourselves when we hit a wall in personal growth: *This is just who I am.* We treat our habits, emotional triggers, and familiar limits like a finished portrait—signed, framed, and unchangeable. But modern neuroscience offers a gentler and more liberating truth. The human brain is not a rigid machine. It is a living landscape, constantly reshaped by experience.

Like a tree that survives a century of storms by continuously turning its leaves toward the sun, the brain has a living edge—an ability to adjust, to reroute, to let go of what no longer serves, and to grow in a new direction when the old one becomes cramped or costly. This adaptability is called neuroplasticity. It does more than explain how we learn. It means we can participate in our own becoming. We are not fixed statues. We are works in progress—capable of profound, intentional change.

The brain is often the most familiar system in the body and the least understood. We know it as the command center: receiving information, interpreting it, coordinating movement, emotion, memory, and meaning. We associate it with identity itself. And because it has carried us this far, we tend to trust it implicitly—as though every thought is reliable, every instinct wise, every reaction inevitable.

But the brain is not designed to be right in the way we wish it were. It is designed to be efficient. It is designed to keep us alive.

The human brain contains more than eighty-six billion neurons—cells that communicate through electrical and chemical signals. Those neurons do not act alone. They form pathways and networks: repeated routes of communication that become quicker, stronger, and easier to use over time. Most brains share the same general architecture, but no two are identical. Genetics matter. Life experience matters. What you have practiced—consciously or unconsciously—matters.

Think of a Japanese maple tree growing in a wide, open field. Its branches can stretch outward evenly. Light is plentiful. Space is generous. The tree grows symmetrically because it can. Now imagine that same tree planted in a crowded yard beside a chain-link fence. In that environment it may twist, climb, and lean. It may wrap around obstacles and reach toward narrow openings where sunlight slips through. Its roots may stretch unevenly toward the only reliable water source. It may look lopsided or knotted from the outside.

But crooked trees do not grow crooked to be difficult. They grow crooked to survive.

Human brains are like this. Environments, priorities, wounds, repeated stressors, and emotional patterns all shape the "direction" our neural growth takes. And because building new pathways requires energy, the brain prefers the routes it already knows. Familiar reactions become fast. Old conclusions feel automatic. Even when a response hurts us, the brain may keep choosing it—not out of malice, but out of efficiency. It is easier to walk the well-worn trail than to cut through dense forest.

This is why change can feel so difficult. You are not weak for struggling to shift. You are working against a system that was designed to conserve effort and reduce uncertainty. The brain often chooses what is familiar over what is healthy—not because it cannot change, but because it resists spending energy unless it believes the investment is worth it.

And yet—here is the hopeful part—the brain is not trapped by its own habits. It has a remarkable capacity to reorganize. Neuroplasticity is the brain's ability to strengthen what is repeated, quiet what is neglected, and recruit new routes when old ones no longer function.

When certain neurons fire together repeatedly, their connection becomes more efficient—signals travel with less friction. With repetition, the brain strengthens that route—reinforcing synapses and improving the speed and reliability of the signal. The pathway becomes easier to enter and harder to ignore. It can feel like "this is just how I am," when in reality it is simply what you have practiced the most—sometimes without realizing it.

And the opposite is also true. What is not used begins to fade. Like a tree that sheds branches that no longer receive light, the brain "prunes" pathways that are no longer reinforced. It reallocates resources. It makes room. Both trees and brains share this wisdom: they do not hold onto what no longer brings life—at least not forever.

So the real question becomes: How do we guide this growth?

Not everything about brain development is conscious. Some patterns are laid down early, before we have language for them. Some are born from necessity: ways we learned to stay safe, to cope, to belong. But neuroplasticity gives us a door back into self-agency. We can influence what gets strengthened by what we repeatedly reward with our attention, our actions, and our interpretation.

The brain's reward system reinforces what it predicts will help us. When an action or mindset leads to relief, approval, success, or even temporary numbness, the brain takes note. It tags the pathway: *Do that again.* And this is where the conscious mind matters. We can begin to shape what we treat as a reward. We can decide—slowly, imperfectly, repeatedly—what we want to reinforce.

Consider the goal of exercising regularly. The odds can feel stacked against you: exercise demands energy, and it asks you to build a new routine. If your mind fixates only on discomfort, the brain will file the experience under *avoid.* But if the mind learns to associate the effort with a deeper reward—strength, stability, stamina, a longer life, a calmer nervous system—the brain begins to cooperate. The habit stops being pure expenditure and becomes a path worth building.

You can also choose intentional actions to reduce friction. You can make the trail easier to walk. Maybe you lay out your running shoes the night before. Start smaller than your pride wants. Track progress in a way that makes growth visible. Tie the habit to an existing cue. Celebrate consistency, not intensity. None of this is "cheating." It is strategy. It is working with the brain's design instead of shaming yourself for having one.

When we feel stuck—stagnant, reactive, circling the same physical or emotional ruts—the brain offers us a different story: you are not permanently trapped in the shape you took to survive.

Perhaps childhood wounds taught you to harden certain parts of yourself. Patterns in past relationships may have trained your nervous system to scan for danger. Perhaps a season of scarcity taught you to hoard control. These are not moral failures. They are adaptations. They are the crooked trunk that got you through the storm.

But survival is not the only goal of life.

Now it may be time to grow in a new direction. To prune an old way of thinking that once protected you, but now limits you. To step away from comfort and familiarity in search of a healthier path. And yes—parts of you will resist. Resistance is not proof you're doing it wrong. It is proof you are doing something new.

The rush of anxiety before a difficult conversation. The nausea before a leap of change. The instinct to retreat into old patterns because they feel predictable. Uncertainty can be frightening. Building a new path costs energy. But the very discomfort you feel may be the signal that growth is happening—that your brain is being asked to form new connections, and it is learning, slowly, how to do so.

Maybe it looks like this: you pause with your hand on the doorknob, feeling the old script race ahead—*don't bring it up, don't make it worse, keep the peace.* Your stomach tightens. Your chest gets hot. And for a moment you do nothing—not because you're weak, but because your brain is protecting you the way it always has. Then you take one slow breath, and you choose a different sentence than the one you've always used. Not a perfect sentence. Just a truer one. That is neuroplasticity in real time.

So let's revise the phrase we began with: *This is just who I am.*

In one sense, it's true. You are who you are. You have grown this way for a reason. There is no shame in the twisted bark of habits that helped you endure drought and damage. Honor yourself for surviving.

But who you are now does not have to be who you remain. Change is rarely swift and effortless; it is more often a quiet return—one choice, repeated, until the new path feels like home.

You have the hard-won ability to practice a new way of being until it becomes more natural. You can strengthen what brings life. You can release what no longer does. You can recycle old momentum into new direction. The brain is not a prison. It is a garden, a trail system, a living tree—capable of change, capable of renewal, capable of surprising growth toward the sun.

If all you can do today is notice the old trail and pause before you take it, that counts.

And if you choose growth with intention, your flourishing may become a quiet inspiration—proof to someone else that change is possible, too.

(If you would like a practical companion to this section, *Atomic Habits* by James Clear offers an accessible framework for reducing friction and reinforcing the identity you're trying to build.)

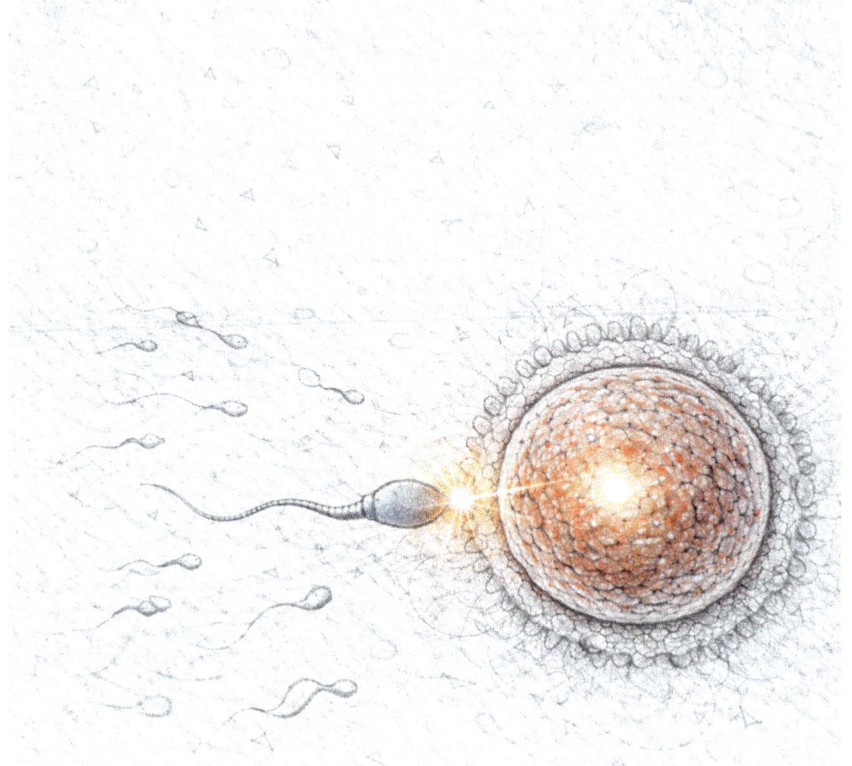

Reproduction:

Creation Requires Vulnerability

Reproduction: Creation Requires Vulnerability

Creation is not a tidy act. Whether it is the creation of new life, a new relationship, a new vocation, or a new version of yourself, it requires something most of us resist: exposure. The reproductive system is the body's clearest proof that life does not emerge from perfect control or complete safety. It emerges from brave participation—an opening that does not deny risk, but learns to hold it wisely. The body prepares. It times. It safeguards. It accepts that to create anything living is to accept the possibility of pain, because growth stretches what once felt sufficient. And it reminds us that creation is rarely a solo act. It is sustained by complementary work—initiative and receptivity, offering and receiving, strength and responsiveness—different roles moving toward one shared outcome. The reproductive system is not merely about making life. It is the body's lesson that what is worth creating will change you, and that vulnerability is not the cost of failure, but the price of becoming.

The human reproductive process is remarkable in a singular way: no other system can transform the body so thoroughly, so quickly, and for so long. From the earliest moment of conception, pronounced and prolonged change becomes necessary to sustain pregnancy and nurture growth through every phase. An entire internal world shifts and stretches to make room for what did not exist before. Pregnancy is rarely described as comfortable or easy—but many would still call it valuable, meaningful, and worth the cost.

Preparation for conception begins long before it takes place. In the female reproductive cycle, hormones rise and fall in a rhythmic pattern that coordinates two kinds of readiness: the development of an egg and the preparation of the uterus. As hormone levels increase, the uterine lining thickens, blood flow increases, and the environment becomes nourishing—ready, if needed, to receive. Then a surge triggers ovulation: a mature egg is released and begins traveling toward the uterus, open to fertilization along the way.

The stage is set—but the window is brief. Most eggs remain viable for only 12 to 24 hours after release. That limited opening is not a failure of the system; it is a boundary. It reflects a wise economy: this much preparation demands energy, and the body does not hold itself in maximal vulnerability indefinitely. It opens intentionally—not without boundaries, but with boundaries that can open.

And conception, by nature, is collaborative. Sperm are surprisingly sensitive to their environment; temperature, pH, and fluid conditions matter, and survival can be brief without the right support. In addition, the reproductive tract is not a neutral hallway—it is part of a living body with defenses designed to protect. And yet, in the right conditions and timing, the body can become welcoming enough for sperm to travel to the egg. When one succeeds, the egg changes almost instantly, altering its outer layer to prevent additional sperm from entering. It is a kind of discernment written in biology: an ability to receive, and an ability to close—both in service of protecting what has begun.

Once fertilization occurs, the zygote divides rapidly as it completes its journey to the uterus, where it will implant and grow. From here, the body's work becomes relentless and intimate. Hormones shift again. Blood volume increases. The immune system adapts, balancing protection with tolerance. The placenta forms as a bridge—an exchange point where oxygen and nutrients can be delivered and waste removed, where two lives remain distinct and yet deeply connected. A quiet reciprocity unfolds every day: sustaining new life while also sustaining the one who carries it.

As pregnancy progresses, the mother's organs reorganize and compress, muscles carry additional weight, and the body does double effort—maintaining its own stability while supporting someone else's development. Pains, cramps, nausea, fatigue, headaches—many of these can be commonplace. Growth can be uncomfortable when boundaries expand and new strength is required. Yet discomfort is not always a sign that something is wrong. Often it is simply the sensation of making room.

Perhaps the most profound embodiment of this truth is labor. Waves of contraction build and return, again and again—pressure that can be intense, disorienting, and consuming. The cervix dilates far beyond its usual limits to create an opening where none existed. And as the baby emerges, nothing will ever be the same for both mother and child. The mother's body has been changed permanently in response to her new identity; it is not a clean transition, but a real one. Her mind is reshaped by responsibility. Her child becomes both great joy and challenge—an ongoing invitation into the long work of care. The child will mature and grow into their own person, moving further into independence with each season. They will venture into the world and live out meaningful experiences of their own. And the mother has the privilege of looking on with pride while knowing that by creating new life, she has created something new within herself too.

Vulnerability is often mistaken for recklessness—as though it means throwing open every door and hoping nothing breaks. But the body models something wiser. It creates with boundaries: conditions, timing, and discernment. It opens intentionally, not impulsively. That is what emotional maturity looks like, too—choosing what you will allow in, and what you will not, without sealing yourself off from life. Whether you are creating a relationship or a project, neither can thrive without the right measure of authenticity and openness.

One of the quiet miracles of reproduction is that it requires partnership—not necessarily romance, but cooperation. It takes offering and receiving, signal and response, seed and soil, protection and yielding. A balancing act of reciprocity. These are not "male" and "female" virtues. They are human roles that show up everywhere: in parenting, in friendship, in teamwork, in healing. Some seasons ask you to initiate—to speak first, to reach out, to offer what you have. Other seasons ask you to receive—to let yourself be helped, to be influenced, to be changed. A life that can only give becomes exhausted. A life that can only receive becomes stagnant. Creation requires both.

We tend to interpret discomfort as a warning that we should stop—especially if we have been hurt before. And it is true: not all pain is sacred. Some pain is a boundary being crossed. But the reproductive system tells another story alongside that one: discomfort is not always danger. Sometimes it is stretching. Sometimes it is the body making room for what it has decided is worth sustaining. Creation often hurts—not because it is wrong, but because it is real. The pain is not a punishment. It is proof that something inside you is changing shape.

So when you find yourself longing to create something—new trust, new intimacy, a new path forward—remember the body's wisdom. It does not demand perfect safety before it begins. It prepares. It discerns. It opens anyway. It accepts the stretching as part of the process and honors recovery as part of the cost. And it refuses the myth of solitary strength, insisting that life is sustained through exchange—through giving and receiving, offering and being changed. Creation requires vulnerability—not because vulnerability is easy, but because it is the only way life continues to unfold.

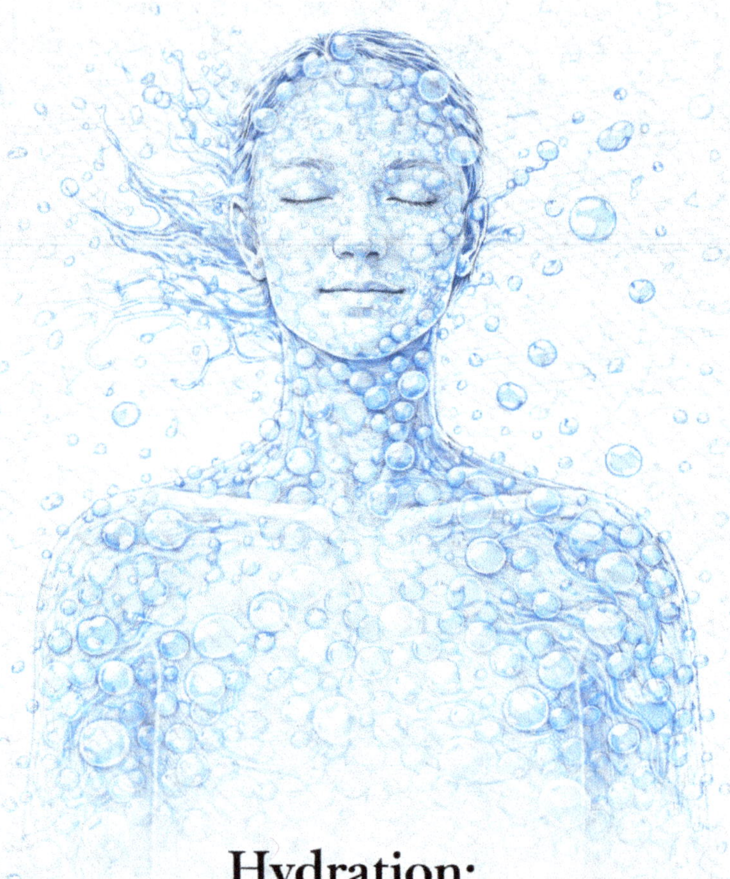

Hydration:

Remember What You Are Made Of

Hydration: Remember What You Are Made Of

Even after all of our discussion thus far, we have yet to touch on the most foundational essence of the human body—something that connects the entire organism across every system. It is impossible to live without, and yet many of us neglect it regularly.

Water.

It composes roughly sixty percent of the human body. It is the most basic building block of life as we know it—not just human life, but all life. Water carries nutrients and oxygen. It regulates temperature. It cushions organs and allows systems to communicate. Without a steady supply, cells wither, circulation slows, and balance is lost. Its importance cannot be overstated. It quite literally makes us who we are.

And yet, many of us rarely treat water as a priority. Perhaps because it seems abundant, we forget how essential it truly is. But when the body is deprived of hydration, everything suffers. Waste accumulates. Energy fades. Thinking becomes cloudy. Fatigue, dizziness, and confusion follow. The kidneys strain. Momentum is lost. Like a stagnant swamp, a dehydrated system cannot move forward—it cannot renew itself.

By neglecting what is most basic, we quietly lose access to our own strength.

Throughout this book, we have explored many lessons the body offers—some calling for action, others for rest, reflection, or release. But before any of that can take root, there is a simpler remembering required.

Remember what you are made of.

Safety. Love. Purpose. Self-worth. These are not luxuries. They are foundational. Without them, even the most sincere effort will feel exhausting and unsustainable. But when they are present—when they are replenished—clarity returns. Strength follows.

So let's begin here.

You are loved.
You are wildly strong.
You can do hard things.
You are allowed to make mistakes.
You are never alone.

Thank you for letting me sit with you for a while, my friend.

About the Author

Matthew Tamer is an oncology pharmacist practicing in a hospital setting, where science and humanity meet every day. His work has given him an intimate understanding of the human body—its resilience, its fragility, and the intricate systems that sustain life. It has also placed him alongside people navigating some of the most profound emotional moments of their lives, from fear and loss to hope, meaning, and connection.

Through years of clinical practice and personal reflection, Matthew has come to believe that the body is not merely a biological machine, but a source of quiet wisdom. Each system carries lessons about balance, adaptation, and care—lessons that extend far beyond physiology.

At the core of his life and work is a commitment to living with intention. He believes that life offers insight in every moment, whether ordinary or painful, and that wisdom often reveals itself when we slow down enough to listen. This book was written as an invitation to do just that.

www.ingramcontent.com/pod-product-compliance
Lightning Source LLC
Chambersburg PA
CBHW070821260726
48660CB00005B/1938